Clinical Practice Development Using Novice to Expert Theory

Barbara Haag-Heitman, MS, RN, CS
Aurora HealthCare
Milwaukee, Wisconsin

AN ASPEN PUBLICATION®
Aspen Publishers, Inc.
Gaithersburg, Maryland
1999

Library of Congress Cataloging-in-Publication Data

Clinical practice development using novice to expert theory /
[edited by] Barbara Haag-Heitman.
p.   cm.
Includes bibliographical references and index.
ISBN 0-8342-1247-1
1. Nursing models.   2. Clinical competence.   I. Haag-Heitman, Barbara.
[DNLM: 1. St. Luke's Medical Center (Milwaukee, Wis.). Nursing Division.
2. Nursing Service, Hospital—organization & administration.
3. Clinical Competence.   4. Nursing Theory.   5. Peer Review, Health Care.
WY 125 C641 1999]

RT84.5.C57   1999
362.1'73'068—dc21
DNLM/DLC
for Library of Congress   99-15859
CIP

Orders: (800) 638-8437
Customer Service: (800) 234-1660

About Aspen Publishers • For more than 35 years, Aspen has been a leading professional publisher in a variety of disciplines. Aspen's vast information resources are available in both print and electronic formats. We are committed to providing the highest quality information available in the most appropriate format for our customers. Visit Aspen's Internet site for more information resources, directories, articles, and a searchable version of Aspen's full catalog, including the most recent publications: **http://www.aspenpub.com**
Aspen Publishers, Inc. • The hallmark of quality in publishing
Member of the worldwide Wolters Kluwer group.

Editorial Services: Joan Sesma
Library of Congress Catalog Card Number: 99-15859
ISBN: 0-8342-1247-1

Printed in the United States of America
1   2   3   4   5

Table of Contents

**Chapter 5—Determining Staff Nurses'
Developmental Stages Using
a Peer Review Process** **87**

Jeanne Smrz DuPont and Barbara Haag-Heitman

Chapter 6—Coaching: An Integral Component . . .**117**

Alice Kramer

Contributors

Patricia Benner, RN, PhD, FAAN
Professor of Nursing
Department of Physiological Nursing
University of California, San Francisco
School of Nursing
San Francisco, California

Richard V. Benner, PhD
President
Benner Associates
Berkeley, California

Laura J. Burke, PhD, RN, FAAN
Director of Nursing Research
Nursing Research Center
Aurora HealthCare-Metro Region
Milwaukee, Wisconsin

Carol Camooso, RN, MS
Professional Development Coordinator
Center for Clinical and Professional Development
Massachusetts General Hospital
Boston, Massachusetts

Theresa Dirienzo, RN, BSN
Staff Nurse
Preadmissions Test Center
St. Luke's Medical Center
Milwaukee, Wisconsin

Jeanne Smrz DuPont, RN, BSN
Staff Nurse
Emergency Department
St. Luke's Medical Center
Milwaukee, Wisconsin

Marie P. Farrell, EdD, RN, MPH
Walter Schroeder Endowed Chair in Nursing Research
Aurora HealthCare-Metro Region
Professor of Nursing
University of Wisconsin
Milwaukee, Wisconsin
Adjunct Professor of Nursing
Harvard School of Public Health
Boston, Massachusetts

Vicki George, RN, MSN, PhD
Vice President
Chief Nurse Executive
Aurora HealthCare-Metro Region
Milwaukee, Wisconsin

Sharon Gray, RN, BSN
Nurse Clinician
Sinai Samaritan Medical Center
Milwaukee, Wisconsin

Barbara Haag-Heitman, MS, RN, CS
Aurora Health Care
Milwaukee, Wisconsin

Alice Kramer, RN, MS
Clinical Nurse Specialist
St. Luke's Medical Center
Milwaukee, Wisconsin

Nora Ladewig, RN, MSN
Clinical Nurse Specialist
St. Luke's Medical Center
Milwaukee, Wisconsin

Sue Luedtke, RN, MSN
Patient Care Manager
Surgical Cardiac Unit
St. Luke's Medical Center
Milwaukee, Wisconsin

Susan A. Nuccio, RN, MSN
Clinical Nurse Specialist
St. Luke's Medical Center
Milwaukee, Wisconsin

Tim Porter-O'Grady, EdD, PhD, FAAN
Senior Partner
Tim Porter-O'Grady Associates
Assistant Professor
Emory University
Atlanta, Georgia

Julie Raaum, RN, MS
Family Nurse Practitioner
Milwaukee Adolescent Health Program
Milwaukee, Wisconsin

FOREWORD

Often during times of great change, the foundation upon which one constructs an approach to life or work is shaken. The chaos of the vortex of activities, which indicates the myriad kind and number of changes, can often be overwhelming. Without a clear notion of the conceptual and contextual framework for one's life and work, the meaning that sustains each of us can get lost.

Nursing as a discipline is struggling with a loss of meaning. In this time of great change in health care, much of the context that defined the milieu in which nurses work has been altered dramatically, affecting the activities and functions of nursing practice. The hospital, once the bulwark of the health care enterprise, is now becoming something else, and much of what was expected of nurses there is now shifting to other constructs and to other providers. There is nothing so threatening and unsettling as the belief that what nurses have to offer is no longer understood or even desired in the emerging practice environment.

The centrality of the role of the nurse has helped define the work of the profession. Those nurses however, who defined themselves in the context of what they do now find themselves without definition and are floating across the shifting sands of health care service. The result: great discomfort and noise as nurses react to the loss of locus and value and try to save what little is left for them in a transforming health care system.

The challenge in this time for nurses is to realize that what they do is a reflection of who they are. There is much more to the definitive character of nursing than simply an attachment to the various functions and processes that indicate nurse's focus at any given time. Technology is always at work, changing the circumstance of our lives and altering the requisites of work and contribution. Nurses should not expect that they will do the same things forever and that time will somehow protect them from ever changing what they do.

The question for every nurse is: Who am I and what do I have to contribute to the obligations of my profession and the needs of those we serve? Increasingly, the answer entails focusing on mobility, ambulatory services, health scripts, continuity across the lifespan, life management issues, and focus on the health of the community. All of this must now unfold within the constraints of ever more defined financial and performance parameters. Furthermore, there is growing demand for evidence of value and focus on outcomes measures and performance factors, creating an expanding body of knowledge regarding what works and does not as it relates to assuring health and addressing approaches to treating and caring for the sick.

Clarifying core values and processes must now be a large measure of the contribution of nurses to health care. What is that unique value and contribution nurses make in the health continuum that enumerates their contribution to health and health care? How do nurses tell their story and what are the common elements that can be clarified and codified as central to the role of the nurse and the delivery of health service? And just as important, what competencies result from the determination of value that transfer into all clinical situations and verify and validate the real value of nurses in the delivery of health services?

It is these issues that engage the time of nurses in their preparation for the future of health care. The novice-to-expert continuum so well articulated by Dr. Patricia Benner is one of the more powerful vehicles for delineating that value and contribution. In the progressive narratives of nurses' experiences and thoughts around patients and clinical work are the common themes that inform nursing practice and the role of the nurse. Elucidating the stages of development and maturity of the nursing mind and subsequent action helps extend the value of practice and serves to clarify those components of nurse's work that articulate good practice and expert performance. Expectations around assuring that consumers and other providers are clear about what to get from nurses are imbedded in the exemplars that name nursing best practices and contributions.

The strength of this book is the focus on both format and process that evidences workable circumstance for a novice-to-expert framework for competence determination and advancing nursing practice. The depth of thought and conceptual consistency throughout their work attest to the sustainability of the novice-to-expert approach imbedded within the Clinical Practice Development Model created by St. Luke's Medical Center in Milwaukee, Wisconsin. Along with the shared governance structural model, this nursing staff has exemplified commitment to the advancement of nurses and nursing practice for some time now. In this work they show with a high level of clarity how these approaches can be structured, how they work, and the issues that they raise for the profession and the individual.

A growing focus on outcomes will accelerate the demand for a clear relationship of process to the results to which they ostensibly lead. Ultimately, each discipline will need to give evidence of its contribution to the health outcomes of the people and communities they serve. Through the Clinical Practice Development Model, the authors have embarked on a process that will extend the work of connecting process and outcomes for nurses. This will contribute to establishing a clearer foundation for nursing practice and will assist in building into all levels and arenas of practice some common elements and activities that best exemplify the role and contribution of nurses to the health of the community. A side benefit will be the creation of a framework for the mature and professional relationship between nurses and a better way to define the character and content of that relationship.

These are exciting times for health care and for nurses. The challenge for all nurses is to be willing to embrace the opportunity for redefinition and change in role. Through the strategies, processes, and structures outlined in this book within the context of the Clinical Practice Development Model, some of the key elements of the work of preparing nurses for the future are mapped out. This work provides a seminal opportunity to advance nursing practice and value and contributes significantly to forming the foundation for the future of nursing practice.

Tim Porter-O'Grady, EdD, PhD, FAAN

Acknowledgments

No book can be authored without a tremendous amount of background support and activity from others. The encouragement to begin publication of this work grew out of my collegial relationship with Marge Hart and Kimberly Hopey in Pittsburgh, Pennsylvania. They created the first prospectus and facilitated the publication agreement. Thank you both for your inspiration. The thoughtful review and editing support from Patricia Benner, Richard Benner, Marie Farrell, and Laura Burke helped raise the quality of this book and was much appreciated. Tim Porter-O'Grady contributed both advice and insight into the publishing process, which was marvelous—thank you. The preparation of this manuscript was achieved through the unending commitment of Marlys Boyer. Her attention to detail and her energy were both tremendous and I am very appreciative of her contribution.

This work is dedicated to the staff nurses at St. Luke's Medical Center, who shaped the Clinical Practice Development Model through your stories of practice, and to the staff, clinical nurse specialists, and managers who provided the leadership necessary to achieve this monumental accomplishment. I am sincerely and deeply grateful to you all. It was my privilege to help convey your story to others.

INTRODUCTION

Over the past decade the Nursing Division at St. Luke's Medical Center in Milwaukee, Wisconsin, has been guided by three prevailing frameworks: shared governance, novice to expert, and the learning organization. Our shared governance model has evolved with the organization over the years to emphasize decision making at the point of service. Our promotion model, called the Clinical Practice Development Model (CPDM), is based on the Dreyfus Model of Skill Acquisition and the novice to expert framework developed by Dr. Patricia Benner. The learning organization was the most recently introduced framework into our practice setting, and its influence on practice and the culture is emerging.

The CPDM was actualized in the context of the shared governance accountabilities. We believe this grounding phenomenon provided the foundation for sustainability of CPDM amongst competing organizational initiatives and priorities inherent in these times of leadership changes and the like. Much of the writing done for this book was authored by our staff nurses. They were instrumental in creating both the CPDM framework and processes to attain and sustain this change by fully utilizing the power and authority residing within their shared governance councils. Because of the sustaining influence that our shared governance structure has related to the CPDM processes, it is detailed in the Appendixes.

This book describes our organizational journey in the implementation of a staff nurse peer review and advancement model based on a novice-to-expert framework that is grounded in a narrative methodology. Using the day-to-day stories of nurses as the basis for promotion and peer review enhances the opportunity for lifelong learning. Our process fosters the development of learning relationships among staff and nursing leadership, providing the foundation for formation of a learning community, which is vital to the well-being of our organization.

Glimpses into possibilities for an interdisciplinary model and adaptation to a multi-hospital system are also provided.

Chapter 1

Vision to Reality: A Historical Perspective

Nora Ladewig and Julie Raaum

To believe in something not yet proved and to underwrite it with our lives; it is the only way we can leave the future open.

— Lillian Smith

Over the past decade we have experienced tremendous transformation in our practice and culture as staff nurses at St. Luke's Medical Center (SLMC) in Milwaukee, Wisconsin. We believe we have achieved empowerment for decision making that affects our practice at the point of service across the care continuum. We have done this by working with the nursing leadership in redesigning our promotional model and by applying it within an accountability-based shared governance structure. The movement from a traditional career ladder into a clinical practice development model (CPDM) was a pivotal change that contributed to our success. But these and other changes did not occur easily. Our success with the development and implementation of the CPDM into practice and culture at SLMC was realized through the progressive and visionary leadership demonstrated by our chief nurse executive and emulated by our nursing staff, managers, and clinical nurse specialists. A common vision of commitment to excellence in patient care and partnership was evident in this leadership group. As a result, empowered nurses grew to value their clinical learning and caring practices in new ways, and began to make their clinical knowledge and caring practices more visible and accessible. Our journey from the old paradigm of the career ladder to the new paradigm of the CPDM occurred almost simultaneously with our transition to an empowered model of shared governance. Our need to gain knowledge and skill to work in both models opened us to great learning, accelerated our positive growth as a nursing division, and dramatically began to change our culture. A timeline illustrating our transition is located in Appendix A.

FROM CAREER LADDER TO A CLINICAL DEVELOPMENT MODEL

I was elected Practice council chair during the transition to a true accountability-based shared governance model. One of our first priorities as a new council was to develop a compatible promotional and developmental framework that would live and breathe the true essence of our practice, which was reflected in our new conceptual model. The vital concepts of quality, caring, accountability, holistic care, and collaboration would need to be closely woven and integrated into the new model. Dr. Patricia Benner's work on novice to expert, using nurses' own stories to reveal their practice wisdom within their developmental level, appeared to offer a solid and practical start. We were surprised at how the narratives were able to make visible the complexity of our clinical judgment and caring practices. This was the start of our journey into a new era and we are continually evolving our practice and shaping our future.

Courtesy of Jim Leichtle, RN
Staff Nurse, Diagnostic and Treatment Center

REFLECTING ON THE PAST

The power of using narrative descriptions of practice to capture the complexity of clinical judgment and caring practices is demonstrated in a story from a St. Luke's staff nurse. She submitted her narrative, which was used in her peer review, to the

American Association of Critical Care Nurses, and as a result received their "Excellence in Critical Care Practice Award."

Discharge planning was part of my daily practice, but I was really put to a challenge when I met Marie and her husband Tom. I was new to the CV group as a clinician and the other nurses had all had their "turn" managing her discharge. It wasn't a surprise that Marie was admitted again with a bout of CHF; it was her third admission in as many months. I sensed everyone involved in her care had become frustrated and it was my turn to do the discharge planning. The doctor thought a "new perspective" might help.

So here I was, meeting them both for the first time only a week before the planned discharge date. I knew I had my work cut out for me when I first walked into her room. Marie was a beautiful but frail woman of 75 years. She certainly didn't look her age, but her chronic illness showed in her eyes. She barely tipped the scales at 100 pounds, and it was easy to guess that her nutritional status was poor. "I can look at all her objective data later," I thought. First I had to get some direction from her and Tom.

They were hesitant to talk with me at first. I was an unfamiliar face. And why was I there "when Sandy discharged me last time?" she asked. That was my cue and I decided to be honest with her. "A fresh perspective," I told her. She shared with me all of her trials at home, how long each lasted and how she was readmitted. She had very fragile cardiomyopathy (idiopathic) and "tipped over the edge" if the wind blew her, she joked. At least she's maintained a sense of humor, I thought. That's important. I stopped her short of reading back her medical records to me and asked her and Tom to "tell me something that's not in the records." At first I could tell they were puzzled, but I continued to explain that I needed to get to know them and their needs, what was important to them and what she wanted to do when she went home. It wasn't long before they began to talk to me about their garden, Tom's pride and joy. And he enjoyed having Marie there to help him, even if she could only sit in the yard and keep him company. They never had children. Marie explained that she had "hundreds" of them, though. She went on to tell me that she had been a schoolteacher and considered each child a part of her. "I gave part of me to each of them," she told me. I was impressed by that thought. I could picture her as a teacher and a good one at that. She had a lot of stories to tell about life.

We talked some more and soon I learned that Tom prized himself on how well he took care of Marie. That was important to him and he felt he had failed by her repeated hospitalizations. He was meticulous about her care, medications, and diet. He tended to her every need. I took the opportunity to do some basic teaching about her disease process and how, despite the best medical management, she could still go into failure. Marie and Tom had a good grasp of her condition and the prognosis. She was not a candidate for transplant because of her age. She made it clear that she did not want to spend her last days in a hospital. She "hated hospitals" and didn't want to die in one. She wanted to be at home with Tom.

Marie knew "what a catch" Tom was. He was so good to her and it was evident the love they had for each other. I wanted to come up with a plan that would help keep Marie out of the hospital and out of failure, not an easy task. I scheduled to meet with them on a daily basis to discuss discharge plans and I offered that I would have some ideas for them tomorrow. As I left the floor I struggled for a clue as how to approach her case.

First I reviewed her charts (volumes). I searched for some ideas. Like most patients with cardiomyopathy, Marie did well while she received inotropes. She had already suffered some end organ damage, with her baseline creatinine approaching 2.0 on admission. Her protein and albumin levels were low and she was malnourished. She suffered from passive right sided failure and ascites that left her feeling full and without an appetite and chronically constipated. The constipation aggravated internal and external hemorrhoids that often ruined a good day for her.

Next I met with the social worker, who gave me some indications about Marie's insurance coverage and different home care agencies that had been involved in her care. I mentioned some of my thoughts for discharge, which were at first met with raised eyebrows.

Finally, I met back with Marie's doctor. He seemed impressed by my knowledge of her in such a short period of time. Unfortunately, he was not impressed with my ideas for discharge. "Home inotropic therapy was meant as a bridge to transplant," he told me. "Marie is not a candidate for transplant, Lori. What benefit will she get from that?" I argued my case with him. Her past records showed that she responded to Dobutrex within 2–3 days. At that point, she was often free of dyspnea and rales and did not require oxygen. Over the course of time she often shed 5–10 pounds of water weight and her appetite and energy level improved. I had researched the cost of home therapy versus hospitalizations every month and the savings would be phenomenal. Most of all, it would allow Marie to be where she wanted—at home. I had pulled a literature search regarding the use of home Dobutamine therapy for Dr. S. to read. Admittedly, all focused on the use of the agents as a means of maintaining a patient waiting for transplant. There was no discussion about the patient wanting to go home to die. He would give it some thought overnight and "get back to me tomorrow."

I was paged the next morning at 8:30 a.m. and Dr. S. asked me to come to his office. "Here comes the letdown," I thought as I walked back to the office. I felt frustrated, as I was not prepared for an alternate plan for Marie at this time. But to my surprise he was willing to give it a chance. "One month," he told me. If she did not show evidence of positive response we would have to try something different. I was elated. Next I had to discuss the idea with Marie and Tom.

I arranged to meet with them in the afternoon. I arranged for the nurse from the home IV company to meet me at the hospital about an hour after my scheduled appointment with Marie and Tom. I was pretty sure they would accept the plan.

It didn't take long to convince them. It met all the requirements they gave me. Marie would be at home, Tom could continue to care for them, and if all worked well, Marie would be able to stay out of the hospital. They were somewhat impressed and surprised when the IV nurse came to visit. I think they felt some comfort in the fact that I was organized and working toward the anticipated discharge date. How could I forget it? Marie reminded me every day that we "promised she could go home toward the end of the week." Her smile was infectious when she teased.

We spent the majority of the day making plans. A Groshong catheter had to be placed and I was given permission to contact the surgeon if Marie and Tom agreed to proceed. The line would be placed the next afternoon. "Perfect," I thought. I could get all the discharge teaching completed by then. The IV nurse returned the following day to discuss how her therapy would proceed. I enlisted the help of the Oncology CNS to assist with central line care home instructions. I learned a few things, too, while sitting in on the session.

Tom was beaming a big smile when he completed his first central line dressing change at the hospital. He was not intimidated at all by the task. He fumbled a bit with the gloves. He had lost a few tips of fingers in an industrial accident years ago, which made some of those fine tasks a challenge.

Finally, I convinced Dr. S. that another gastrointestinal (GI) consult was necessary for Marie. The hemorrhoids had become a constant source of irritation for her. She had to sit up the majority of the day to breathe comfortably and she was often miserable. She was seen in consultation the day before discharge, the hemorrhoids were cauterized, and she was placed on a regimen of stool softeners and bowel stimulants. Marie verbalized to me that she was glad this was finally addressed. She hesitated to complain about them (hemorrhoids) because they seemed so "petty" compared to her other problems. The dietitian met with them prior to discharge to instruct Tom and Marie on a high-fiber, high-protein, high-calorie diet. Again, Tom listened intently, as he did most of the cooking. "You can eat some of my home-grown carrots," I overheard him saying to Marie. There was that smile again.

I met the expected discharge date and the IV nurse would be meeting with them the following morning to begin the Dobutrex therapy. The nurse would meet with them every Monday, Wednesday, and Friday, which were the days planned for infusion. When Tom and Marie felt comfortable with it, they would be given the responsibility of infusing the medication, too.

I made phone calls to them daily at home. I wanted everything to go well for them and it became part of a daily routine. We would make small talk about Marie's condition, but most of the time Tom wanted to tell me of his accomplishments with her care. He reported what he cooked for dinner, her weight, blood pressure, and pulse. He told me how her breathing was and what pills she took so far. To my surprise one day, Tom had me paged at work. I panicked when I heard his voice. He had never called me and I feared that something terrible happened. Not to worry, I was told. Tom just wanted to share his pride in the fact that he had completed his first Dobutrex infusion completely by himself. I felt so good when I hung up the phone. This was going to work.

The month passed and Marie and Tom had an appointment with Dr. S. A check-up of sorts, on all of us. I had kept Dr. S. informed of Marie's progress on a daily or every other day basis. She stayed at her dry weight the entire month, and her lab work looked great! She even had a creatinine of 1.4, a record for her! I was just as impressed as Dr. S. was.

The therapy continued and Marie stayed out of the hospital and out of failure for six months. She succumbed to pneumonia that winter. But she spent the summer with Tom out in the garden. She would sit in the lawn chair while Tom gardened and they talked.

I attended Marie's funeral at Tom's request. There was no greater satisfaction than the smile on his face when he saw me come into the room. He was not bitter over her death as I expected he might be, rather so pleased with the quality of time he had to spend with her.

Courtesy of Lori Hislop, RN, BSN, CCRN
Thoracic Transplant ICU,
St. Luke's Medical Center

An understanding of the present relies on the knowledge of the past. SLMC instituted a career ladder for clinical advancement in the early 1980s. The nursing process was the framework used in this advancement model to describe and characterize nursing practice. In addition, nursing tasks and functional roles were defined and measured as the nurse progressed "up the ladder." The ladder consisted of four rungs or arms: direct patient care (practice), teaching/learning (education), leadership/coordination (management), and research. Over time, the nurse was expected to gain work experience and seniority in this nursing system of delivering care. Generally nurses progressed upward; however, movement downward on the ladder was possible and did occur. They advanced through the first three levels of the career ladder by meeting all care competencies listed at each level. At the fourth level, however, each nurse declared an area of expertise from one of the four arms of the ladder. Competencies at the fourth level varied according to the arm selected and reflected the highest level attainable for nurses remaining in bedside positions (see Figure 1–1).

THE PEER REVIEW PROCESS

Peer review played a part in this career ladder advancement system. The promotional process began when a nurse applied for promotion and had his or her application approved by nursing management. Management approval was the signal for the nurse to begin compiling materials that verified achievement of

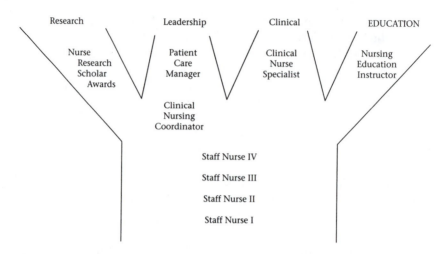

Figure 1–1 St. Luke's Medical Center Career Ladder
Source: Courtesy of St. Luke's Medical Center, Milwaukee, Wisconsin.

an expected level of competency. The applying nurse then validated the petition for promotion. The career ladder peer review panel of two staff nurse peers and the unit manager met to review the nurse applicant's materials and to approve or disapprove promotion. The nurse who was being reviewed and the manager selected the staff nurse members sitting on these peer review panels. At this time, there were no competency measures to evaluate the nurse's ability to participate in the peer review process. Further, no mechanism existed to develop the staff nurse's skills essential for processing and receiving feedback in a peer review forum. Thus, panel members were often selected based on their relationship with the nurse being reviewed, and the process became known as the "pal review."

A LANGUAGE NEEDED FOR PRACTICE

It soon became evident that the nurses who selected the direct patient care arm of the ladder had the most difficult time documenting their expertise in a measurable way. The criteria in the direct patient care tract applied to few behaviors that could be measured quantitatively, despite its comparable worth to the other three tracts. Nurses found it difficult to describe their expertise in delivering care to patients. The evaluation system lacked a language that described the delivery of clinical nursing care regardless of the staff nurse's level on the career ladder, experience, or competency. The career ladder model quickly evolved into one with high performance expectations and low recognition of the unique skills and contribution that each nurse brought to the workplace. The majority of the staff felt that the actual patient care they delivered was not recognized or rewarded in any way. It seemed that the essence of our work was invisible to much of the organization. Not surprisingly, it was during this same period that nursing staff satisfaction with the work of nursing hovered at an all-time low.

THE EFFECTS OF CULTURE ON CARE

The culture and core values of St. Luke's during this period contributed to lack of recognition and reward for direct patient care. New staff were subjected to an orientation process that was lengthy and focused on preparing the nurse to manage any and all aspects of patient care. After orientation was completed, little effort was directed toward helping nurses grow in their ability to provide care to patients.

With no specific efforts directed towards self-growth, nurses looked elsewhere for recognition. A popular method used to gain recognition was to work in a unit that was viewed in a favorable way by the majority of the nursing or medical staff in the hospital. The career ladder perpetuated the way nurses defined themselves as a collective of individuals in specialty departments and exclusive units. Nurses came to know and identify themselves not by who they are, but by the tasks performed and the patient populations they served.

The reality of this environment was that we did not articulate in a universal language the nursing practice that was held in common across the organization. We had come to define and describe ourselves by our differences and specialties rather than by our similarities.

DOING VERSUS BEING

The problem with this distinction was evident, for example, in the progression of patients through the system. Because each unit viewed its uniqueness as positive and sometimes powerful, no coordinated effort was made to assure that the patient and family navigated smoothly through units seen as less important or powerful. Long reports and other delays in transferring patients from one area to another were commonplace. It was not unusual to have information and personal materials important to the patient and family lost in the transfer from one area to the other. This, among other outcomes, created patient dissatisfaction. Without a universal language and focus on a common practice framework, it was impossible to develop and document systems and processes that optimized patient care across the continuum.

By the late 1980s, the career ladder evaluation system had become a "paper monster" and the nursing staff viewed it as a source of great dissatisfaction. The staff criticized it for its complexity and lack of relevance to clinical practice. This level of dissatisfaction prompted the need to find a mechanism for determining meaning and value for nursing practice.

In 1989, the Nursing Peer Review Committee (a group of nurses who reviewed the advancement ladder regularly) prepared to address the nursing staff's dissatisfaction with the career ladder and advancement process. In anticipation of sweeping change, information was gathered internally from the nurses using the ladder and externally from other large hospitals that had a clinical model of advancement in place.

The Peer Review Committee subsequently distributed a house-wide survey to staff and management for feedback. A majority of the staff participated in the survey and this majority's voice was loud, clear, and focused. Common themes identified in the comments were a perceived lack of integrity in the application of the evaluation mechanism between units, a sense of "falling outside of the practice behaviors" itemized in the advancement ladder, and being compensated for nonpatient care professional activities rather than for direct patient care activities. This was succinctly put by one respondent: *"I feel strongly that peer review does not place a strong enough emphasis on the nurse at the bedside. We have placed too much emphasis on committee work and lost the part of what nursing is really about."*

To expand our knowledge, the Peer Review Committee investigated the documentation on clinical advancement programs solicited from six hospitals of similar size with existing nurse peer review components. The committee looked at the programs, at the process used for advancement and peer review, and finally at staff satisfaction with the current process. It was at this time that the work of Dr. Patricia Benner came to our attention and the possibility of using a novice to expert framework for advancement was raised.

SHIFTING THE PARADIGM: IMPLEMENTATION OF A NEW GOVERNANCE MODEL

The 1990s and New Leadership

With the hiring of Vicki George as the new chief nurse executive (CNE) in the early 1990s, the nursing division began a redesign aimed at creation of a work environment that promoted empowerment through professionalism. She facilitated establishment of a professional practice environment that fosters clinical excellence and involves staff participation in the organizational decision-making process. A major redesign in the shared governance model—from an administrative model of participatory management to an accountability-based model of shared decision making—was begun with consultative support from Dr. Tim Porter-O'Grady.

A Majority of Mind

One of the first changes the nursing staff made was the reorganization of the shared governance model into one that integrated nursing management and staff in a true accountability-based system. The new governance system relinquished the multiple, larger-group information-sharing structure for small decision-making bodies called councils. A ballot of peers determined membership of these councils. The first paradigm shift began when the cultural norm shifted from nurses *having* information to nurses *using* information to make accountability-based decisions that would shape and change the way nursing conducted its work.

The new model structurally unified the nursing division into a whole systems framework and began to reframe in new ways nurses' thoughts about the nature and context of their work. A shift in the locus of control and accountability for patient care resulted from this change and the staff developed a new philosophy (Exhibit 1–1) and a new conceptual framework for nursing practice (Exhibit 1–2, and Figure 1–2). The elements of redesign are clearly shown in the framework that underscores accountability, quality, and caring—the components central to direct patient care.

The nursing staff who were the elected members of shared governance councils understood that they would be held accountable for the decisions they made for the nurses they represented in the organization. The staff nurse experience of owning the authority as well as the accountability for decisions was certainly a new one that the CNE clearly supported. The opportunity to have a positive effect on nursing practice was embraced by the newly elected staff leadership. Strategic initiatives were readily designed and implemented with new enthusiasm and commitment. In contrast to the previous shared governance model, decision making was efficient, effective, and powerful to bring about and sustain change. This represented a major shift in our way of doing business. Communication of these changes challenged us as a system.

There was also a gap between knowing about the decisions and having a deep understanding of how these changes would affect both an individual's practice and the practice environment as a whole. In a way, we could think of ourselves as novices in our new governance system and naive to the nuances that would reveal themselves over time. The nursing staff at large displayed little response to the early decisions the

Exhibit 1-1 St. Luke's Medical Center Philosophy of Nursing

St. Luke's Medical Center is a private, non-profit health care center and member of the Aurora Health Care System. People who require a high degree of technological support for the diagnosis and treatment of their health problems look to St. Luke's as a leader in health care. Their health care needs are addressed in a dynamic, ever changing environment that is characterized by personalized care and service.

Nursing practice at St. Luke's Medical Center is accountability based and committed to the delivery of quality care. It is comprised of the care provided by professional nurses as well as the care delegated to others. Authority for clinical decision-making is determined by education and experience along a continuum of novice to expert practitioner.

Caring is central to nursing practice at St. Luke's Medical Center. It mandates a holistic approach to practice. This is actualized through collaboration with the person, their significant others, and members of the health care team both within and beyond the institution. The final outcome of nursing practice then is the attainment of well- being as it is possible, within each person's potential.

Source: Courtesy of St. Luke's Medical Center, Milwaukee, Wisconsin.

elected councils made. For example, identifying councils and council accountabilities, nursing goals, and a conceptual framework seemed to many to have little or no effect on them or their work at this time. This may have misled the shared governance leadership to view the staff's response as one of approval of these new activities and decisions, when perhaps they were not yet really appreciating the effects of these changes.

Implementing the CPDM was the opportunity for our revised nursing shared governance membership to fully explore and exercise the accountabilities within each council (see Appendix B for a detailed description of each council's accountabilities). This exploration of the new governance model and accountabilities revealed that full staff participation was necessary and

Exhibit 1-2 Conceptual Framework of Nursing Practice

Conceptual Framework of Nursing Practice
The conceptual framework identifies the critical elements of nursing practice at St. Luke's Medical Center. It describes what nursing practice is and how it is carried out in this institution.

ACCOUNTABILITY is the ongoing responsibility that professional nurses have for their clinical practice. It is promoted through an integrative shared governance model. It is exercised through enactment of the St. Luke's Medical Center Standards for Nursing Practice. Accountability involves the retroactive review of decisions made and actions taken to determine whether or not they were appropriate.

QUALITY care is nursing practice that is dynamic and individually directed toward the achievement of a mutually acceptable outcome.

CARING is an ethic, a feeling, a way of knowing. Caring means that persons, events, projects, and things matter to people. Because of caring, nursing practice creatively uses diverse strategies to meet a person's unique health care needs.

A **HOLISTIC** approach to nursing practice considers the person as a physical, psychological, social, and spiritual being in continuous interaction with their environment.

COLLABORATION is a process which recognizes, respects, and integrates the perspectives of others to provide quality care.

The integration of these five concepts form the conceptual framework and make nursing practice at St. Luke's Medical Center unique. The level of integration, or the ability to influence the outcome of care is determined by the knowledge and experience of the practitioner.

Source: Courtesy of St. Luke's Medical Center, Milwaukee, Wisconsin.

the option for nonparticipation associated with the previous model would cease to exist. The creation and implementation of the new CPDM (the model development and structure are described in Chapter 3) facilitated a greater understanding of the interconnectedness of the nursing division. "It was the start

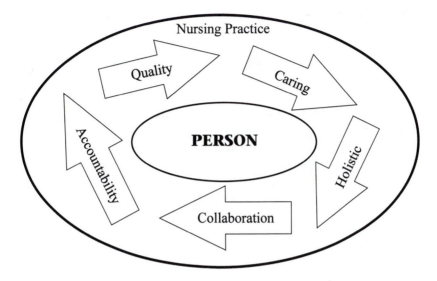

Figure 1–2 St. Luke's Medical Center Conceptual Framework Model
Source: Courtesy of St. Luke's Medical Center, Milwaukee, Wisconsin.

of something going in the right direction," according to one staff nurse.

Redefining Competencies for Nursing Practice

In the transition period from one governance model to the next, the need persisted for a relevant clinical advancement program. In fact, redesigning a clinical promotion program was a priority in the order of business of the new governance councils. This activity was the catalyst for testing organizational commitment to the new shared governance model, beginning with the decision the Nursing Practice Council made to define nursing practice based on the novice to expert continuum. As work on the new promotional model progressed, its relevancy for use as a vehicle for improving the orientation, socialization, and ongoing development of all nurses was recognized. Indeed, it was the beginning of a very positive cultural change.

NEXT STEPS

The novice to expert model was chosen because it satisfied both the intent for acknowledging and rewarding advancing clinical practice and it afforded a valid and reliable measurement mechanism of nursing practice. Benner Associates served as consultants. Their expertise about this theory of skill development in nursing helped staff and leadership develop a greater appreciation for what is not measureable by conventional processess. Chapter 2 presents details of Benner's work, which provided the foundation for the new clinical practice development model that was to follow at St. Luke's.

Chapter 2

The Clinical Practice Development Model: Making the Clinical Judgment, Caring, and Collaborative Work of Nurses Visible

Patricia Benner and Richard V. Benner

> People should think things out fresh and not just accept
> conventional terms and the conventional way of doing
> things.
>
> —Buckminster Fuller

A complex social practice such as nursing requires attentive caring relationships with patients and families, professional commitment to develop practical knowledge, astute clinical judgments across time about particular patients and families, and good collaborative relationships with others on the health care team. All of these practices are more variable and relational than can be spelled out in or mandated by discrete lists of tasks and objectives. In other words, they cannot be managed by the usual managerial approaches to standardization and control. They require professional practice with dedicated professionals who have a strong internal and collective sense of good practice and a commitment to be good practitioners. Sometimes the practice may be completely routine, with no surprises or unusual demands. But when a patient's vulnerability, criticality of illness, or breakdowns in the system of care occur, good practice and the system must rely on intelligent dedicated professionals with front-line knowledge and responsibility—knowledge professionals who solve problems and take needed actions to ensure the safety and well-being of patients and their families. Such a practice is often superogatory, meaning that it goes beyond the call of duty or lists of tasks and of routinization. A static control and command type of management falls short of capturing the relational and practical wisdom of the clinician. Indeed the best of such a practice is often hidden from the standards and protocols that attend to what can be routinized and managed in the practice.

Nursing practice is centrally concerned with making astute clinical judgments, skillfully performing and timing nursing and medical interventions, engaging in caring relationships with patients, and working collaboratively with other health care team members. These four main areas of nurses' skilled know how all occur within relationships with particular patients, families, and other health care team members, occur across time, and require timing. Because they are contextual, temporal, and relational, they remain invisible to most descriptions of nursing practice and the usual industrial engineering task analyses of a nurse's work. These judgments of skillful and relational aspects of nurses' work cannot be standardized yet they encompass major areas of clinical knowledge development and experiential learning within the organization.

Because the nurse is a knowledge professional who works with the patient and communicates and collaborates with other health care team members on behalf of the patient and family, much of the experiential learning and practical wisdom within particular organizational contexts resides with the nurse. Yet, it is precisely this knowledge that may remain elusive and invisible within the organization. Usually, little is done within organizations to capture the experiential learning and practical knowledge of the nurse so that it becomes collective and cumulative. Tasks analyses, information management tools, such as the nursing process and proficiency checklists about technical procedures, although relevant to nurses' work, fail to capture the relational and judgment aspects of nursing that are so central to good nursing practice. Consequently, when checklists related to tasks are used as measures of the nurse's performance, the nurse's central role is trivialized because clinical judgment with particular patients and relational work are rendered invisible by discrete lists of objective tasks. As a result, much of the moral and relational work of the nurse is overlooked and remains unsanctioned and invisible, with little or no organizational processes and structures designed to reflect this central work. Furthermore, much experiential learning and local institutional wisdom are lost.

The invisibility of nurses and their practice has permitted miscalculations about effectiveness and reliability that nursing knowledge work brings to hospital-based practice. Only the lack of understanding of the centrality of the clinical judgment role of nurses in maintaining patients who are critically ill, nursing them back to health, and easing their suffering, have permitted unattuned reductions and replacement of registered nurses to occur. Miscalculations about the role of nurses will continue until their work is made more visible to the structures and processes of the organization. Organizational decisions affecting nursing that do not understand and take into account the importance of strong clinical practice and its development in terms of impact on the patient and impact on the effectiveness of the overall organization will, in time, cause the organization to suffer the loss of both patients and finances.

Over the last 20 years, we have been working with hospitals to help nurses see and learn from their practice, both as individuals and as a shared practice within particular hospital settings. Three aspects of nursing practice are made visible through this developmental and interpretative approach. First, the practice becomes visible to the individual nurse as the nurse has the means of reflecting on his or her own practice. Because there is little public language or official sanctioning of the central nursing functions of clinical judgment, skilled interventions, caregiving work, and clinical leadership of a diverse health care team, these functions are poorly recognized and accounted for in the formal organizational structures and processes. Consequently these nursing functions are pushed to the margins and are usually considered as a part of the "informal organization." Second, the practice becomes visible to nursing colleagues so that experiential learning and clinical knowledge become public, and therefore, collective and cumulative. Third, the larger system in which nursing practice occurs becomes visible in terms of nursing's contributions to the organization and in terms of the organizational supports and impediments to good nursing practice.

The Clinical Practice Development Model (CPDM) is designed to capture and extend these less visible but vital aspects of nursing practice of clinical judgment, caring, and collaboration. In order to do this, strategies that include peer review and nurse's own experience-near narrative accounts of their practice with particular patients and families are required (Geertz, 1983). An experience-near narrative includes the narrator's concerns, perspectives, and experiential learning. It includes chronology and dialogue, and is told and written in the first person voice. It is essential that a command and control managerial approach not be used in these areas that are fraught with risk and high variability, and that are strongly conditioned and influenced by organizational constraints, resources and demands. The first condition of the CPDM is that a climate of openness and trust is established and that the focus is on developing the practice as a socially organized endeavor made up of individual humane knowledge workers with a shared vision for practice.

In order to make the collective reflection on practice effective, it was necessary to impact three levels: the personal, the peer group, and the system. We discovered in our work with a number of hospitals that nursing groups often take the concepts from the book *From Novice to Expert* (Benner, 1984) and apply them in standard and formal ways using the terms and levels of skill acquisition in an abstracted form, creating statements that were thought to reflect the concepts without strong links to practice. Often nursing staff and administration attempted to quantify the statements in a checklist and scoring form to determine practice level. The results of the decontextualized approaches did not capture the complexity or the relational nature of clinical nursing practice. This approach leaves out context, the temporal flow of events, clinical and ethical reasoning about particular patients, and collaborative work, which is incongruent with the original research on skill acquisition and clinical judgment (Benner, 1984; Benner, Tanner, & Chesla, 1996; Benner, Hooper-Kyriakidis, & Stannard, 1999). The underlying methodology of the Novice to Expert research was narrative based and observational. The richness and complexity of practice, both individual and collective, is missed by checklists of skills, regardless of how the skills are described. Often the form took the familiar nursing process descriptors, with a small quantity of the process skill described at entry level and more of the same process skill later on. Our research consistently found qualitatively new skills and abilities and new organization of the understanding of practice with experiential learning over time.

Based upon this persistent misunderstanding, we began working with St. Luke's Medical Center in Milwaukee, Wisconsin, and other hospitals over a longer period in order to train the staff in reflectively reading nursing narratives. The consulting occurred over the course of a year with at least four on-site visits from the consulting group. Because the methodology and process differs from traditional approaches, the consultants coached and instructed nurse peer groups and administrative groups in the use of the narratives to reliably evaluate practice levels and to articulate new areas of clinical knowledge. The consultants' goal is to help nurses discover the local and specific knowledge and clinical wisdom in nurses' practice.

At St. Luke's, the narrative work group developed the descriptive CPDM based upon reading many narratives from throughout the hospital. The skill of reflecting on and interpreting narratives is based upon knowledge of clinical nursing, but guidance is required to learn to read the narrative within the bounds set by the narrator, and to identify the relevant concerns that organize the narrative. The time spent on reflecting on actual clinical nursing practice has many pay offs. The process itself enhances collective clinical inquiry and knowledge development. Reflecting on practice levels and describing the local experiential wisdom enriches the vision of nursing practice in local settings. The collective reflection on practice instills pride and creates new imagination for developing practice.

Clinical practice is a socially embedded knowledge that draws on theoretical and scientific empirical knowledge but also on the practical know how, compassionate meeting of the other, and front-line knowledge work of practitioners. As Polanyi (1958) points out, good clinicians always know more than they can tell. The practitioner, whether nurse, lawyer, teacher, or social worker, reasons about the particular across time, observing transitions in the client's condition, and also transitions in his or her own understanding of the clinical situation. Nurses, like other practitioners, work in complex social environments. They work in collaborative teams that collectively achieve what cannot be achieved alone by any one practitioner. Part of the practical knowledge of practitioners has to do with communicating their understanding of patient transitions and their own transitions in clinical grasp across time to other team members (Benner et al., 1999). Clinicians' practical knowledge also includes understanding how the social system works in their particular organization. For example, how to get the most timely responses from other departments, when to get another clinical consult, or seek advice on evaluating a clinical situation. Unlike pure science that can exert extensive (though not perfect) control over the conditions of the scientific experiment, the clinician's knowledge is situated and unfolding as the patient's clinical condition changes. Clinical knowledge is necessarily ambiguous and requires interpretation. This is why good clinicians seek to strengthen their clinical judgments by consulting with other clinicians, so that pooled experiential wisdom and differing perspectives can improve clinical judgments and fill in missing information (Benner et al., 1996). Also, nurses must clearly communicate their clinical understandings to other nurses, who are caring for the client when they are not present, as well as to other disciplines on the health care team.

This picture of the practical wisdom required to be a good clinician is complex enough without considering the relational work of caring for others during times of vulnerability. Nurses and physicians cannot be mere technicians, applying their craft to inert objects, but must engage in collaborative relationships with patients and families that are based upon trust. This relationship is fiduciary, meaning that the clients' best interests are protected even when clients cannot speak for themselves (Benner, 1997; Sharp, 1997). Caring practices are central to nursing practice. Caring practices involve more than connection or concern with the other, they require skilled know how about helping and advocating for vulnerable others in the contexts of cultural diversity and complex organizations. In our study of critical care nurses we found that the skill of involvement was central to becoming an expert clinician (Benner et al., 1996). If nurses did not learn how to be engaged and attentive without being overwhelmed or over-identified with their patients and patient's families, then their ability to learn from clinical experience was greatly hampered (Rubin, 1996).

Complex systems are designed to create safety through redundancy and routinization, so that steps and procedures are designed to limit human error and lapses in attentiveness. Nursing and medicine are practiced in large and complex bureaucracies that require such systems of routinization. This kind of system design and improvement is based on system checks and reinforcements for attentiveness. But such systems, although necessary, are not sufficient. The complexity and risks of nursing and medical care require knowledge professionals who can solve problems on the spot. The relational nature of the work calls for skills of involvement (Benner et al., 1996; Benner et al., 1999). Noticing changes in the patient's condition and unexpected turns are based upon engagement and skilled know how that comes from cumulative experiential learning about usual trajectories of illness and usual responses to therapies as well as potential deviations and potential problems. Effective delivery of patient/family care requires collective attentiveness and mutual support of good practice embedded in a moral community of practitioners seeking to create and sustain good practice. Such a moral learning community cannot claim or expect infallibility, it can only promise to address system failures and structures that impede good practice, and to close knowledge and practice gaps that contribute to poor practice. This vision of practice is taken from the Aristotelian tradition in ethics (Aristotle, trans. 1985) and the more recent articulation of this tradition by Alasdair MacIntyre (1981), where practice is defined as a collective endeavor that has notions of good internal to the practice. Even though one may not be able to spell out all ways the notions of good practice may be realized, the participants in the practice (practitioner and client) can recognize instances of good and poor practice as fitting in a broad vision of practice. Such a collective endeavor with shared meanings and notions of good works in spite of the impossibility of articulating all the elements that make up complex human practices that require ongoing improvement and innovation. However, such collective endeavors must comprise individual practitioners who have skilled know how, craft, science, and moral imagination, who continue to create and instantiate good practice. Excellent practitioners can contribute to system design and supportive infrastructures but more importantly they breathe life into these systems.

Narratives of such a practice are a gift both to the narrator and to those reading the story because they are not individual "productions" but are rather stories of relationships formed in the context of caring for the ill and vulnerable. This is why the narrative workgroup and clinicians had to develop a climate of mutual respect and confidentiality in which risks and disclosures involved in writing narratives could contribute to learning and growth. As the CPDM evolved, making the experiential learning of nurses visible, clinical judgment, relational, and collaborative work became more apparent. The institutional impact of making the judgment, caring, and collaborative work visible had enormous side benefits in terms of clinical knowledge development and informal learning between nurses reflecting on everyday practice. Also, focusing on improving the institutional climate for such practice continues to unfold.

It is a mistake to map onto professional nursing practice a contractual vision of explicit tasks and duties carried out in predictable and stable circumstances. If the practice could be carried out in this mechanical and predictable fashion, then knowledge workers or professionals would not be needed. Good management in a mixed professional and bureaucratic organization (Blau & Scott, 1962) has the conflicting responsibilities of developing systems that routinize reliably what can be predicted and standardized while creating an environment of responsibility and problem solving in highly variable, complex situations. Highly variable complex work requires developing dynamic learning climates where knowledge workers are empowered to go beyond the standard requirements and redesign work structures and processes, based upon experiential learning. This is how practitioners develop cumulative wisdom. Such bureaucratic systems must attend to the life world of the professional community and encourage the relational work required by caring for vulnerable others, and empower professionals to advocate for the patients/families' best interests.

The CPDM assumes that usual practice of practitioners is facilitated or constrained by the design of the system. And although practitioners may overcome the impediments and constraints of the system much of the time, the ceiling of their usual practice is enabled or impeded by the structures and processes of the organization and work climate. The goal of management is to encourage best practice. Therefore, reading of narratives is a respectful process that looks at the ethical and clinical concerns of the practitioner in the context of the situation where levels of staffing may have been inadequate, or the knowledge supports may have been missing. The focus is on how to design the system so that best practices flourish. Practice resources and constraints related to good and poor outcomes are examined.

The CPDM seeks to open up the clinical knowledge of the practicing nurse so that other nurses can benefit from their blending of experiential practical wisdom so that collective and cumulative wisdom can be developed in a learning organization (Senge, 1991; Benner et al., 1999; Brykczynski, 1998). This experiential wisdom includes capturing the clinician's skilled know how in advocating for patients in local specific systems. The CPDM is not a remedial or even a normative system in that it is not designed to detect knowledge of standards and protocols or even the latest scientific knowledge. Therefore, it cannot replace systems for updating and evaluating scientific and technical knowledge. The CPDM is designed to maximize the clinical learning of practicing nurses and continuously improving the design of the system. In this way, good practice and experiential learning are reflected in re-design, and practical learning associated with adopting new science and technology is captured and communicated.

Because developing clinical expertise is based on experiential learning, the practitioner at each stage of the model can be the best practitioner at whatever stage—best beginning practitioner, the best possible competent level practitioner, and at the proficient and expert stages, be astute at recognizing the unexpected and subtle deviations from normal. At each stage of skill acquisition, all practitioners can be engaged in working out new experiential wisdom. Experiential learning is not based upon mere passage of time but on openness to learning. Experience is the turning around of preconceived notions or recognizing a poor grasp of the clinical situation (Benner, 1984; Benner et al., 1999). What is not possible or reasonable is to expect clinicians to practice beyond their own experience level with any particular patient population. For example, a clinician who has seen only one open heart surgery patient recover cannot be expected to make qualitative distinctions or comparisons with other recovering open heart surgery patients. This ability to compare between whole concrete clinical cases is distinctly more nuanced and more powerful for recognizing deviations from the usual course than is captured in textbook descriptions or critical pathways. This is an obvious statement but it is often ignored in a technical vision of practice, where it is imagined that critical pathways and protocols can make explicit the myriad trajectories and variations in practice. Nevertheless, clinicians cannot be held accountable for what they have not had the opportunity to learn in their practice. But they can work in a collaborative climate where the collective goal is to make the best use of the experiential wisdom of one's colleagues and all experiential learning.

Likewise, it is not possible to mandate that anyone "care" or engage in caring practices. Caring practices are based upon meeting and responding to particular concrete others (Benner, 1997). It has been my (Patricia Benner's) teaching practice to use first person experience-near narratives to uncover knowledge embedded in clinical practice. The students are asked to write first person, experience-near narratives about clinical situations that taught them something new about practice or that stood out in their memory for other reasons, such as mistakes made, lessons learned, or examples of the best of their practice. The criteria for evaluating the narrative are clarity, vividness, honesty, and providing the reader with enough detail to be able to imagine the situation. Consequently students may write about breakdown situations vividly and provide reflective commentary on a narrative that is thoughtful, and receive a good grade.

One year in a class of 70 nursing students five stories from neonatal and pediatric intensive care nurses were about caring for an infant where the infant or child had died and the nurse came to question her level of grief over the death. These nurses were often the ones who knew the premature infant in the illness context more intimately than the parents, and therefore had been in the position of helping the parents come to know the child. Invariably these narratives asked questions such as the following:

- Did they cross boundaries of involvement that they should not have professionally crossed?
- Did they get over-involved because they felt the loss of the child so keenly when the child died?
- Was it reasonable to expose oneself repeatedly to loss?
- How could they protect themselves?

We concluded that no one could ever demand that they care for an infant to the point of engrossment and suffering over the loss of the child. This is beyond the call of duty and can never be mandated. From an ethical obligation perspective, the most anyone can ask is that the nurse is gentle, attentive, and respectful of the infant and parents. No one can demand that they love the infants because such a demand would be supererogatory (Benner, 1997; Vetlesen, 1994). And yet an ethical violence is created if nurses do not ever become engrossed in the infant to the point that they know the infant in his or her particularity. Such engrossment inevitably leads to a sense of loss when the infant dies.

These nurses assisted in the social birth and social recognition of the infants as fellow human beings. These social recognition and relational practices humanize the clinical environments of neonatal critical care units (Benner et al., 1996). There would be no social traces left of the infant if the nurses did not come to know the babies and even to love them, and coach the parents in coming to know their infants in these foreign biomedical environments. This is indeed a challenging call made by an ethic of care—to acknowledge that we cannot within a rights and justice framework, order, command, or mandate that nurses care for these infants—and yet acknowledge that a great ethical violence is created if the nurses do not care. Without the nurses' caring relationships with these particular infants and parents, neglect instead of responsiveness to the infant and parents will occur. Articulating a social and personal ethic that cannot be mandated or legislated, but the absence of which creates ethical violence, neglect, mis-recognition, and abuse, is indeed a challenge in this era of economism, individualism, and commodification of health care. It does not fit a managerial command and control model. As psychologists have taught us to more clearly articulate, there are many ways to get caring practices wrong, such as burnout, co-dependency, and heroic helping, or even blaming the victim (Benner, 1998).

Because excellent diagnostic, monitoring, therapeutic interventions and caring practices are relational and contextual, the clinician is unsure whether such excellent practice could occur without particular relationships with patients and families, particular collaborative relationships with physicians and others, particular organizational structures and processes, and even particular timing of the clinical events. Although the technical and scientific aspects of the practice can be formalized in procedure books and critical pathways, the human expertise to orchestrate and carry out the practice cannot be. The nature of expert clinical practice always has this local specific knowledge-event-relationship-context quality about it. It cannot be universalized or standardized. The most one can say is, given the variety of contextual, relational, and timing contingencies, that clinicians who are good clinical inquirers and who have benefited from much clinical experiential learning will do best in these complex open-ended clinical situations. Furthermore, those same clinicians will still be constrained by the level of collaboration, resources, organizational structures, and processes available.

We began our consulting with St. Luke's Medical Center with a focus on narratives throughout the hospital. We found areas of extraordinary strength in care of the family, and also a pervasive practice of clinical forethought, anticipating crises, preventing crises, and preparing the environment for the most likely eventualities (see also Benner et al., 1999). The caring practices were exemplary and widely distributed throughout the hospital. The goal was to infuse these caring, growth encouraging practices into the peer review system. The goal was to keep the focus on the positive capacities and learning tasks of each stage of clinical development. Initially, it was unclear to the staff nurses whether the process was going to be more of a focus on presentation skills rather than on the best of their practice and their own clinical knowledge development in practice. It was here that the shared governance model was essential because the staff nurses did have the opportunity to take up the challenge of making the system equitable and facilitating. They were able to express their fears and participate in designing safeguards in the system such as having coaching available for all nurses, and ensuring that all nurses were interviewed in the peer review process.

As the CPDM developed, the focus was increasingly on experiential learning and developing the practice. The clinical leaders were able to respond to the staff nurse's fears and understandable resistance by responding to the concerns of the clinicians. They also worked on their ability to give direct, honest feedback that did not resort to shame and blame. The feedback focused not only on the clinician's individual performance but also on the resources and constraints present in the organization. The panels stayed within the real structures and constraints of the narratives presented. The goal of CPDM is that no one should go up for a promotion process who cannot achieve the promotion. This is why the coaching is so important. The process is developmental because in the process of going for promotion the nurse reflects on practice and gains feedback on his or her practice in ways that foster growth and encouragement for good practice. Likewise, coaches and peer review panels have opportunities to reflect on the practice as described by the nurses. CPDM is not a remedial system, but an excellence system that should positively reward growth and excellent practice. Through this intensive review process, the caring work, clinical judgment, intervention skills, and collaborative work of nurses became more visible to the formal system so that increasingly public recognition and sanctioned organizational attention to nurses' experiential learning and wisdom were included in system design and re-design.

In the intensive training of the peer review panels, three peer review skills were emphasized.

1. Provide open questions in the interview.
2. Give evaluative comments that reflect constraints and resources in the situation.
3. Articulate the nature of the skilled know how in the narratives.

The overarching goal was to make the peer review process positive, communicative, and provide accurate feedback to clinicians on their practice. Even the most fearful and skeptical nurses came away from the panels feeling that they had been heard and respected for their knowledge and caring work (see Chapter 5). Increasingly, the language of the peer review panels became clearer about notions of good practice, and about resources and constraints in the system supports for good practice at St. Luke's. As the panels became more skillful, they increasingly identified and wrote up re-design considerations that would facilitate or disimpede the good practice evident in the narratives.

USING CLINICAL NARRATIVES TO REFLECT ON PRACTICE—GROWING AND EXTENDING EXCELLENT PRACTICE

Reading Narratives

The use of clinical narratives to uncover knowledge in clinical practice begins with a careful reading of a group of clinical narratives from across the health care organization by persons who have become skilled at reading clinical narratives. These persons learn to reflect on local clinical practices by learning to identify:

- clinical concerns that organize the story,
- clinical judgment as revealed by the unfolding of the clinical situation over time,
- and the caring aspects of the work.

The members gain skill in how to look at practice from the intensive practice of reviewing 50 or more narratives from nurses across the organization. This process gives an increased understanding of local clinical practice as it is supported or hindered by local organizational structures and processes. The individual nurse's practice becomes visible but the commonalities in practice and the institutional aspects of practice also become clearer in relation to supporting or hindering good practice.

In order to describe characteristics of stages in practice, it is ideal to collect narratives from at least two nurses from each unit in the hospital who are experienced and who are considered to be excellent clinicians by peers and supervisors. This group of nurses becomes the narrative resource group for the professional practice committee and can be a resource in a variety of ways for the committee. With this first stage of the CPDM, nurses embark on a self-study of their practice, which includes giving language and examples of the best of their practice. Because first-person experience-near narratives are used, relational caring work, clinical judgment, and coordination of the health care team efforts can be described over time.

This process of the committee reading a collected group of clinical narratives results in at least two outcomes. First, the group begins to identify themes and characteristics of the practice in the local setting. The myriad themes initially identified by the committee are usually reduced through conversation and consensus to three or four areas of strength, which are hallmarks of locally based practice (for example, "strong collaborative practice" or "patient-family centered care").

Identifying Characteristics

Next, under each of these themes characteristics are identified, such as: "Attends to family issues related to the patient's illness." These characteristics are exemplified by at least three narrative excerpts. All characteristics are grounded in actual narrative examples. This is an open-ended process in that new examples can be submitted as this aspect of practice grows and is better understood. This process of illustrating local knowledge about experiential learning, clinical judgment, caring work, and clinical leadership legitimizes that knowledge, making it visible and open to discussion and learning. This is not an abstract description of what might be hoped for as the "ideal" practice, but a careful reflection on nursing as it is currently practiced in the local setting with all the extant resources and constraints. Narratives are also read in relationship to the stages of skill acquisition described by Dreyfus & Dreyfus (1986), Benner (1984), and Benner et al. (1996).

At the same time the committee identifies the positive themes and characteristics of local practice, it also begins seeing, as a natural product of the process, areas where the practice is impeded or blocked. This identification of the problems for the practice opens up, often for the first time, structures and processes that prevent the best nursing practice. For example, a common impediment we often find in hospitals is a lack of collaborative practice between physicians and nurses and between nurses themselves. When a group of narratives written by nurses from across the hospital without any planned focus on the issue of collaboration reveals that collaboration is a widespread problem, it becomes visible and interpretable within the local setting. Such identification of both strengths and impediments of the practice is based on a rich "narrative database."

Through this process, nurses gain skill in looking not only at individual practice, but they learn also to look for system issues in terms of strengths of the practices as well as impediments, gaps, or silences. A cadre of nurses, who have been trained to reflect on practice and to articulate areas of experiential learning and clinical knowledge development, can pass these interpretive skills on to others. The narrative database and increased skills in articulating the knowledge embedded in practice provide a rich learning environment and a knowledge development strategy. Nurses are empowered to publicly present central aspects of their role, which have been marginalized in the past.

Peer Review and Narrative Coaching

The third major component is the use of a peer review system and narrative coaching to help the nurse, writing a set of clinical narratives, to describe and reflect on his or her practice and to be able to discuss practice with peers based upon clinical situations that stand out for the nurse. This moves the reflection, review, and development of practice from managers to nursing peers. This peer-based system focuses on practice and on developing the practice by making more of the experiential learning of clinicians public and therefore available to others. The intention of this approach is to focus on identifying and developing excellence in practice. It does not focus on deficit identification and remediation, which are more fairly and easily handled by the usual paper and pencil evaluation strategies.

Management tools, for the most part, are created to be quick, efficient, easily used paper systems, easily scored, regardless of the user so that numeric results can be compared to others. This strategy works best for identifying knowledge deficits and maintaining standards. The abstracted categories are usually scored by a person in a managerial position who has limited opportunity to see the practice of the person and may be removed from direct patient care. Because these strategies do not assess clinical judgment, timely interventions, and relational work, they address minimal knowledge for basic performance standards. They cannot address excellent practice.

Ethical and clinical knowledge are forms of practical knowledge. They are a thinking-in-action and, therefore, are not just a technical application of knowledge to practical situation. They may also be considered to be productive thinking rather than just subsuming information under categories, or classification (Benner et al., 1999). In nursing and medicine, these forms of practical knowledge are facilitated or impeded by relationships with others. For example, a climate of trust and openness on the part of client and practitioner creates different possibilities for good clinical outcomes. And a climate of distrust can render good practice impossible. Ethical and clinical reasoning are linked because one's notions of good guide what is considered to be a good clinical outcome. Notions of good may differ between patient, family, and clinicians. For example, a patient may prefer mental alertness and therefore limit the use of any sedatives or pain medication, even though pain or sleeplessness may be presenting significant problems for the patient. The patient and clinician must then work out the best strategies to achieve as much pain relief and sedation with as much mental alertness as possible. This illustrates that communication and relational skills are central to good clinical practice.

First person experience-near narratives generated by clinicians allow reasoning-in-transition across time and the relationships between clinicians and patient to become visible and open to reflection (Benner et al., 1999). Such narratives work best when they are created in a climate of safety, trust, and openness. The clinician reveals more than he or she consciously controls, because a first-person experience-near narrative reveals the perspectives and concerns that the clinicians themselves may only dimly perceive. What the clinician considers important to tell and what is memorable to the clinician determine the stories that can be told by a particular clinician with any coherence and detail. Thus, a clinical narrative provides a basis for reflecting on practice that can reveal unnoticed aspects of the clinician's perspectives and knowledge. These unnoticed aspects may reveal experiential learning and clinical wisdom that have never been fully articulated or made visible to the clinician or to others. Blind spots and knowledge gaps can also show up in narratives. Because clinicians are participants and members of a practice tradition with common meanings, expectations, notions of good, skills, and habits, narratives from such a practice discipline are never just individual, independent productions. They are stories of what the practice will allow, what patients/families seek from practitioners, and what the organizational structures and processes make possible. In this sense, it is not only practice that is shared, but also stories from that practice. For all these reasons the narratives of individual nurses must be treated as a reflection not only on the individual's practice, but also on the practice that is possible in a particular organization.

READING AND REFLECTING ON NARRATIVES

The first and foremost requirement is that the narrative is written and read in its own terms. This is the most difficult aspect of narrative methodology to convey, because many people believe that the stories will be so individual and private that no one will be able to make sense of them. So it is usually only after a group has read a number of narratives that they recognize that the narratives are generated within a practice discipline, within a particular organizational culture, and within a specific moral community of practitioners. Stories have a collective quality to them with shared notions of good and shared understandings of good and poor practice. The most common response is that formal criteria must be generated to judge all the narratives from that same formal criteria in order to be fair and just. In the St. Luke's project initially, this took the form of identifying characteristics of practice in great detail at different stages of skill acquisition and the specified domains so strongly that it was difficult at first for some to write and read narratives in their own terms. Fortunately, for the process, narratives are robust and resistant to such constraints, and usually the story of the actual clinical encounter shines through. When the focus is more on "staging" an employee (the old clinical model) than on articulating and extending excellent practice (the developmental model), narratives are glossed over for their particular knowledge and concerns. Consequently, readers and narrators may overlook clinical knowledge that may not have been captured previously. The focus on the organizational resources and impediments to good practice along with re-design implications evident in the narrative can also be overlooked (Benner et al., 1999). Because the peer reviewers share the practice and the organizational context, they can come to the narratives with local understandings. This has both advantages and disadvantages. The advantage is that they can recognize the commonly experienced resources and constraints to good practice. The disadvantage is that they may not see the obvious, or assume that they understand what sounds familiar (e.g., "I gave the patient emotional support.") because they take it for granted. Consequently, there is no substitute for reading the same narrative as a group and comparing interpretation. The following is an example of a training narrative.

Mr. H. was progressing "normally" post-OHS (open-heart surgery). He was between seven and nine days post surgery. I had taken care of him for the past three days on day shift. We had developed a good rapport with each other by the beginning of day four. This day shift started like the others, going into my patient rooms to see how they were doing.

Mr. H. was already up and showered. At first glance, nothing seemed to be abnormal. I completed a physical assessment and began talking to Mr. H. about how he felt and what discharge teaching we could work on that day. Mr. H. wanted to tell me something but he wasn't sure how to describe what he was feeling. After several minutes, I found he was having an intermittent chest clicking sound, especially at night—when people were around it never seemed to happen.

At first I thought about Mr. H's history of surgery one year prior and the conversation we had the first day I cared for him. He had told me that Dr. T. had said that the sternum had never healed completely from the first surgery. Secondly, I assured Mr. H. that I, indeed, did believe what he had told me and was going to inform the surgical team of what was happening, since he had told the PA [physician's assistant] who had assessed him that morning (the PA had been skeptical).

I did re-listen to his heart tones as I had not heard anything prior to my second assessment. I still didn't hear anything. About 30 minutes had gone by when Mr. H. called me into his room because he was experiencing the clicking again. When I listened this time, I heard a very faint clicking. When I left the room, I found the PA who had seen the patient. I informed him of my findings but was informed that my assessment must be wrong. At first, I thought he must be right since I had never dealt with an unstable sternum before. I checked with the charge nurse and questioned her about these findings. I received positive feedback from her that the sounds I described could indeed be an unstable sternum.

I decided to wait for the MD to do rounds and I would make sure that he knew about what was going on (even if I was going to make a fool of myself). Several hours had passed and this patient's click was louder and more consistently present now. I also noted that the incision line was not separating but was "bubbling" in a few spots. I re-approached the PA, who was again on the floor at this time. I received the same "You are stupid" look and brush off with the comment that the "MD is doing rounds shortly."

Within 30 minutes, the MD was on the floor. I followed them into Mr. H's room and listened to them talk about releasing Mr. H. the next day. Mr. H. was not going to say anything, so I needed to speak up. I felt I was putting any credibility I had on the line. I realized being a patient advocate was more important than what someone thought of me. I also knew that I had to start trusting my nursing instincts. I told the MD what I had heard and what Mr. H. had told me. The MD looked at the sternum and listened also. He heard the sternum click and told the PA they were going to have to open the puffed areas to see how unstable it really was. I stayed with the patient during this and offered as much support as I could.

Mr. H.'s stay progressed to about one and a half months. Mr. H. went to the OR and had surgery to tighten wires and debride a sternal infection that had set in. After this situation, I felt that I have more confidence in my physical assessments and I realized how important it is for nursing to stand up and become a patient advocate.

This is a clearly written narrative with the nurse openly describing her experiential learning in (1) recognizing the clinical signs and symptoms of sternal instability and infection after open heart surgery, and (2) learning to advocate for the patient, first with the PA and then with the physician. This nurse demonstrates good clinical inquiry skills and persistence. She states that she has a good rapport with the patient but does not expand on what this covering phrase "good rapport" looks like or sounds like in practice. The fact that the patient trusted her with uncertain clinical signs and worries suggests that she indeed did have good rapport, and that the patient trusted her. She attends and respects the patient's self-report. She has had no prior experience with an unstable sternum, and after not receiving a good hearing from the PA, checks with the charge nurse. Because of imminent patient discharge and the patient's silence, she then speaks up for the patient. She describes this as risking her credibility because she was still unsure of the evidence for an unstable sternum. But she took this risk of having her assessment dismissed or being considered wrong and brought the problem to the attention of the physician. She describes this experiential learning as gaining experience and confidence in advocating for the patient. She states the following: "I realized being a patient advocate was more important than what someone thought of me. I also knew I had to start trusting my nursing judgment and instincts." This is crucial experiential learning. There is no evidence in the narrative that she followed up with the PA to ensure that this opportunity for improving clinical recognition of sternal instability and infection was not missed.

This nurse is skillful at clinical inquiry and an effective knowledge professional. She is clearly competent and demonstrates movement in the direction of proficiency with this narrative. She demonstrates her engagement and commitment to patient advocacy. How can the peer review panel make this clinical inquiry and insight fullness available to other nurses? Review of this narrative suggests questions for the panel interview, for staff development, and for quality improvement.

- Question for panel interview: Does this clinical learning stay personal or is it extended to others, particularly the PA?

- Question for staff development: Could this be a teaching case on post-operative chest surgery complications?
- Question for quality improvement: How often is the incidence of sternal instability and infection after surgery occurring? This question should be forwarded to the Quality Assurance Committee.

The narrative presents an occasion for making good nursing practice visible and rewarded. Experiential clinical learning is expensive and whenever possible should be extended to others in order to develop cumulative and collective wisdom. As more narratives are written and reflected upon, understanding of the local practices increases.

THE DISTINCTIONS, DIS-JUNCTURES, AND RISKS IN USING NARRATIVES AS RESEARCH DATA AND USING NARRATIVES AS EVALUATION TOOLS

Narratives created in a protected, anonymous context of research and interpreted in terms of socially embedded knowledge and skill and narratives generated openly in a social context of evaluating an individual nurse's practice have different social meanings and inherent social responsibilities. Whereas narrators in any context can choose whether to publicly present a particular story from their practice, the consequences for submitting a story for public scrutiny and evaluation for promotion tied to salary increase differ radically from the risks of disclosure and loss of privacy when presenting narratives for research evaluation. A narrative is not under the complete control or mastery of the narrator and may therefore reveal more about the narrator's practice than may be intended by the narrator. In the case of an excellent practitioner, what is revealed offers the opportunity for articulating newly won experiential knowledge or wisdom. In the case of conflicted inter-departmental or intra-professional relationships, a narrative may reveal constraints and impediments to good practice. In the case of conflicted or disengaged caregivers, the narrative may reveal failed interpersonal relationships or a lack of knowledge or skill. If knowledge and skill gaps are found upon working with the narrator, we strongly recommend a coaching process to help the nurse identify problem areas. But we also strongly caution on making the individual responsible for system failures and inadequacies. This creates a standard of hyper-responsibility and allows system inadequacies to continue with the expectation that super-practitioners will overcome chronic system inadequacies and failures. Interpretation of the narrative that focuses only on traits or talents of the narrator and not on the context of practice or the socially structured possibilities for practice in a local setting may cause the nurse unfairly to be held responsible for system breakdowns or failures that may then remain unchallenged.

This was evident in a recent research study with data collection during 1996–1997 (Benner et al., 1999). In this study some work systems had become so de-stabilized by downsizing and short staffing that nurses could no longer maintain a quality of practice satisfying to them. Although these nurses continued to monitor quality and manage increasingly frequent breakdowns in the systems, they were often overwhelmed with the impossibility of managing systems designed to continue to deliver highly technical medical care in the absence of adequate caregiving support (Benner et al., 1999). Clearly the narrators should not be held responsible for disclosing such pervasive inadequacies and failures in the system, but the damage of punishing the messenger is ever present in closed administration systems governed more by cost controls and profit motives than by the essential costs of providing reliable care. In order to prevent corruption and protect the integrity of the use of narratives for self and other evaluation, the process must have multiple safeguards in place. The nurse should have access to adequate staff development and coaching. The goal should be to have no nurse go forward for a promotion that they are unlikely to achieve. The process should be governed by peers outside the nurse's own work group to prevent favoritism, or negative bias. The peer evaluators must be carefully trained to identify the social structures, resources, and constraints that shape the practice described. Peer-reviewers must become astute in recognizing that practice is a socially embedded, shared enterprise and that improvement of practice requires improving the social structures and processes of work, and not just the achievements of individual practitioners. It is unreasonable to expect continual heroic overcoming of persistent system failures and flaws. A developmental approach requires respect and honesty so that individual practitioners can uncover system failures and flaws. The peer-review must be open and dialogical, and not done behind closed doors in the absence of the narrator. It is after all, the jointly held practice of nursing care that is being evaluated and not just the individual nurse. The integrity of the process requires institutional integrity as well as individual integrity.

We recommend a multi-method approach to assessment with the individual nurse presenting. For example, the nurse can prepare a portfolio containing at least three personal narratives from practice along with other relevant evidence such as documentation of her practice, letters of reference from nurse and physician colleagues, peer-observation assessments, and unsolicited patient/family letters. Such a multi-method approach gives the nurse the opportunity to present the fullest range of practice.

The risks are high in a peer-review system that includes narratives generated from practice. However, the rewards of making the central aspects of nursing knowledge and practice visible, the collective attention given to capturing experiential wisdom, and the relation to high-quality patient care and outcomes make this approach invigorating and energizing to those who are willing to take up the challenge of increasing collective and cumulative wisdom within the organization.

REFERENCES

Aristotle. (1985). *Nicomachean ethics.* (T. Irwin, Transl.) Indianapolis, IN: Hackett.

Benner, P. (1984). *From novice to expert: Excellence and power in clinical nursing.* Menlo Park, CA: Addison-Wesley.

Benner, P. (1997). A dialogue between virtue ethics and care ethics. *Theoretical Medicine, 23,* 1–15.

Benner, P. (1998). When health care becomes a commodity: The need for compassionate strangers. In J.F. Kilner, R.D. Orr, & J.A. Shelly (Eds.), *The changing face of health care* (pp. 119–135). Grand Rapids, MI: William B. Eerdmans.

Benner, P., Hooper-Kyriakidis, P., & Stannard, D. (1999). *Clinical wisdom and interventions in critical care: A thinking-in-action approach.* Philadelphia, PA: Saunders.

Benner, P., Tanner, C.A., & Chesla, C.A. with contributions by J. Rubin, H.L. Dreyfus, & S.E. Dreyfus. (1996). *Clinical expertise in nursing practice: Caring, clinical judgment and ethics.* New York: Springer.

Blau, P.M., & Scott, W.R. (1962). *Formal organizations.* San Francisco: Chandler Publishing Co.

Brykczynski, K.A. (1998). Clinical exemplars describing expert staff nursing practices. *Journal of Nursing Management, 6,* 351–359.

Dreyfus, H. E., & Dreyfus, S.E. (1986). *Mind over machine.* New York: The Free Press.

Geertz, C. (1983). *Local knowledge, further essays in interpretive anthropology.* New York: Harper.

MacIntyre, A. (1981). *After virtue: A study in moral theory.* Notre Dame, IN: University of Notre Dame.

Polanyi, M. (1958). *Personal knowledge: Towards a post-critical philosophy.* Chicago: The University of Chicago Press.

Rubin, J. (1996). Impediments to expert clinical practice in critical care units. In P. Benner , C.A. Tanner, & C.A. Chesla (Eds.), *Clinical expertise in nursing practice: Caring, clinical judgment, and ethics* (pp. 170–192). New York: Springer.

Senge, P. (1991). *The fifth discipline.* New York: Doubleday.

Sharp, V.A. (1997). Why 'Do no harm?' In D. Thomasma (Ed.), *The influence of Edmund D. Pellegrino's philosophy of medicine* (pp. 197–215). Dordrecht: Kluwer.

Vetlesen, A.J. (1994). *Perception, empathy and judgment: An inquiry into the pre-conditions of moral performance.* University Park, PA: University of Pennsylvania Press.

Chapter 3

Developing the Clinical Practice Development Model at St. Luke's Medical Center

Barbara Haag-Heitman

I saw the angel in the marble and I chiseled
until I set it free.

—Michelangelo Buonarroti

THE EMERGENCE OF A NEW MODEL

The nursing staff began work on the new developmental model for recognition and advancement in the spring of 1992. From the beginning, nurses were clear on two major issues: recognition and reward for the nurse's work at the point of service, and reliable performance measurements needed to be the foundation of the new process. Exhibit 3–1 shows the contrast between the proposed developmental model and the more traditional career ladder. The model illustrates the thinking of the members of the shared governance team and the nursing leadership members as the organization shifted from the career ladder to the development model.

Under the new governance structure, the accountability for quality patient care and defining all issues and activities related to nursing practice belonged to the Nursing Practice Council (NPC), and the council was responsible for developing the conceptual framework, clinical standards, and criteria for competencies. The NPC subsequently commissioned a group to define

Exhibit 3–1 Development Model vs. Traditional Career Ladder

Developmental Model	Traditional Career Ladder
1. Practice Focused: Movement along the continuum is based solely on clinical practice development.	1. Not practice focused: Movement along career ladder for promotion is predominately based on committee work, teaching and preceptor opportunities, leadership and charge roles, and presentations at care conferences and research activities.
2. Movement is one directional on a continuum from Novice to Expert.	2. Can move up the ladder through promotion and down the ladder through demotion, i.e., transfer to another area.
3. Internally motivated. Advancement through experience and knowledge acquisition.	3. Externally motivated and acquired, i.e., committees, projects.

Source: Courtesy of St. Luke's Medical Center, Milwaukee, Wisconsin.

and describe the practice of the professional nurse along the novice to expert continuum. A steering committee was formed for the management of issues related to the implementation of the new model (Chapter 4).

GETTING STARTED

A Resource Group of experienced staff nurses representing all types of practice settings at St. Luke's Medical Center (SLMC) was formed to establish a broad level of participation in the design of the new model. The majority of nursing units were represented by 33 members, which also included representatives from Clinical Nurse Specialists and Patient Care Managers groups. This group was essential, as it facilitated the collection of staff nurse narratives for use in the model design and served as the communication link with the nurses at large. The Resource Group met with Benner Associates in April 1992. Through Benner's demonstration of the narrative or story telling methodology, the staff began to recognize both the art of nursing and the culture of SLMC. The narrative reflections supported the decision to move away from a model based on tasks and competency based performance to a model more reflective of the unique contribution of nursing as a profession. The staff and leadership also began to identify the organizational changes that were necessary to facilitate excellence in practice.

The NPC commissioned a satellite workgroup out of the Resource Group, and named it the Narrative Workgroup. It did this as it recognized the efficiency and effectiveness of a smaller workgroup to act as the actual design team. The goals of the Narrative Workgroup were to (1) identify different levels of skill acquisition within St. Luke's, (2) distinguish major domains or themes of practice from our current accounts of best practice, and (3) develop the processes and tools for reading narratives. These processes would help identify areas of clinical knowledge, notions of good practice, and caring practices, and aid in developing a reliable way of identifying levels of skill acquisition. The Narrative Workgroup membership represented that of the NPC Council during the time the model was being developed and included 10 elected members, eight of whom were staff nurses who had achieved Level III or IV on the former career ladder and represented specific practice areas. A Clinical Nurse Specialist, a Patient Care Manager, and one ex-officio academic consultant were also members of the NPC. The Clinical Nurse Specialist (CNS) on the NPC led the Narrative Workgroup, which assured linkage to the NPC whose authority it was to approve the work.

NARRATIVE WORKGROUP SELECTION

The CNS put out a call for workgroup members in the usual manner through the nursing newsletter. Volunteers came forth and the workgroup leader made the selection based on the

Exhibit 3–2 Nursing Representation on the Narrative Workgroup Reflecting Membership of NPC

Narrative Workgroup	Nursing Practice Council
1 - Same Day Surgery	2 - Ambulatory Nurses
1 - Emergency Department	
1 - Surgical/Neuro Intensive Care	2 - Intensive Care Nurses
1 - Cardiovascular ICU	
1 - Cardiac Medical	4 - Med/Surg Specialty Nurses
1 - Pediatrics/Women's Health	
1 - Birthing Center	
1 - Postanesthesia Recovery	
1 - Clinical Nurse Specialist	1 - Clinical Nurse Specialist
1 - Facilitator—CNS from NPC	1 - Patient Care Manager
1 - Patient Care Manager	

nurse's area of representation, his/her potential to provide leadership for change, and the probability that the nurse's current practice was at the proficient or expert stage of practice, as Benner's work has defined expert practice. The original Narrative Workgroup consisted of two staff nurses from the Ambulatory area; two from Intensive Care; four nurses from Med/Surg and Specialty units; one Patient Care Manager; and two Clinical Nurse Specialists with the CNS workgroup leader acting in the facilitator role (membership is illustrated in Exhibit 3–2). Each nurse, representing the perspective of nurses in their practice areas, was charged to integrate these perspectives into a whole practice model.

Presently the NPC membership does not mandate representation from specific nursing areas or levels of staff development. This change on the NPC from specialty representation to representation from nursing at large signifies the growth in trust and understanding about collective nursing practice brought about by experience in the shared governance model and shared understanding from the CPDM process.

CONSULTATION SUPPORT

Consultation with Benner Associates supported the Narrative Workgroup process. Their guidance was critical in understanding the novice to expert framework, learning the clinical narrative methods needed to develop the St. Luke's model, and validation of the model throughout each stage of the development process. Early in our process of developing the expert stage, we came upon narratives that did not seem to fit with the rest of the expert narratives. With consultative support we were able to validate our findings and identify the developmental stages that these narratives represented. Making the distinction between the proficient and expert stages was one of the greatest challenges with which they assisted us. Seeing the progression from accurately identifying the region of the problem in the proficient stage to an intuitive grasp of the clinical situation found in the expert stage required more time to learn than the other stages did. Perspectives from their consultants on design and implementation from other sites across the country provided additional insights and direction prior to the time of peer review to the Narrative Workgroup, particularly around the benefits of someone to play a supportive role to the staff during narrative development. The coaching role, which is discussed in Chapter 6, emerged as a result of this discussion. The group also used Benner's book, "From Novice to Expert," along with several related writings to support their work.

FIRST STEPS IN DESIGN

The Narrative Workgroup held its first meeting in May of 1992 following Benner's visit and Benner's educational presentation to the nursing body at large. The charge of the workgroup was to define the practice of the staff nurse along the novice to expert continuum by examining the St. Luke's nurses' narratives. Staff nurses wrote their clinical stories (in the first person) about care they provided to patients and families. No coaching was prescribed as to the content or length of these stories in this first set of narratives. Each nurse had a 10-month time frame to complete the work. The workgroup replicated the qualitative methods, a situation-based interpretive approach that Benner described and used (Chapter 2).

The Narrative Workshop's first task was to develop the Expert framework of practice. Its members spent the first several meetings reading the presumed "expert" narratives the group solicited. As a basis to begin the work, the group made the assumption that the members of the Resource Group represented expert practice, as they had achieved the top levels of the career ladder and were considered experts by their managers. This assumption was supported, but subsequently, not supported fully due mostly to the focus on leadership, education, and research measurements used in the previous model. The narratives were read for their major concerns, areas of clinical knowledge, and notions of the good.

DEVELOPMENT OF PRACTICE DOMAINS

The members further examined the narratives by comparing Benner's domains of practice with the descriptions of practice in the individual narratives. They made notations in the margins of each narrative regarding the domains of practice and other observations, including any impediments to practice that showed up. They noted that over a short period of time not all the presumed "expert" narratives were at the same stage of practice, and those narratives were set aside for future consideration.

Within several meetings, the workgroup grew in their skill at reading narratives. They no longer found it necessary to scrutinize meaning from each narrative line by line; rather, they would read the narrative as a whole and look for broader practice themes. The Narrative Workgroup planned periodic meetings with the NPC, Steering Committee, and Resource Group to report progress and facilitate understanding of the emerging framework, to plan communication strategies, and to engage in dialogue about model design and implementation issues. At one of the early meetings the Narrative Workgroup shared the long list of themes and descriptive statements compiled from the expert narratives. At this time they were exploring how to arrange these statements using practice themes or domains. Through the use of team learning and perspectives of others at the meetings, it was discovered that these statements correlated nicely with the essential components of the Nursing Conceptual Framework (described in Chapter 1). They then organized descriptive statements from each of Benner's seven domains under the three themes from the Conceptual Framework that included Caring, Clinical Knowledge and Decision Making, and Collaboration (Exhibit 3–3). This communication link proved to be critical in developing the model at all stages. Later during implementation, the shared understanding of this larger group helped provide the necessary leadership to facilitate the implementation process.

Following the completion of the expert framework, it was presented to the NPC for their approval. The NPC unanimously endorsed the Expert stage, which is illustrated in the following outline.

CLINICAL PRACTICE DEVELOPMENT MODEL
STAGE 5: EXPERT

Definition

Stage 5 nurses are expert practitioners whose intuition and skill arise from comprehensive knowledge grounded in experience. Their practice is characterized by a flexible, innovative, and confident self-directed approach to patient and family care. Expert nurses operate from a deep understanding of the total situation. They put into perspective their own personal values and are able to encourage and support patient and family choices. Expert nurses collaborate with other caregivers to challenge and coordinate institutional resources to maximize advocacy for patient and family care in achieving the most effective outcomes.

Exhibit 3–3 Comparisons of Domains of Nursing Practice Between the Two Models

Benner's Novice-to-Expert Model	St. Luke's Clinical Practice Developmental Model
• Helping role • Teaching-coaching function	Caring
• Diagnostic and patient monitoring function • Effective management of rapidly changing situations • Administering and monitoring therapeutic interventions and regimens • Monitoring and ensuring the quality of health care practices	Clinical Knowledge and decision-making
• Organizational and work-role competencies	Collaboration

Source: Courtesy of St. Luke's Medical Center, Milwaukee, Wisconsin.

Caring

1. Presencing: Being with the Patient
   a. Establish trusting relationship with patients grounded in a philosophy of "being with" rather than "doing to" a patient. "Being with" is characterized by a mental and emotional presence that evolves from deep feelings for the patient's experience.
   b. Actively listen in an effort to understand, though not necessarily agree with, patient and family choices.
   c. Demonstrate a deep understanding of the unique meaning of health, illness, and disease on a patient and family.
2. Giving Hope and Creating a Healing Environment

a. Promote healing by helping the patient and family cope with the fears and concerns that accompany life changes.
b. Embody a caring attitude and provide an environment of hope and trust in which gentleness and compassion allow for the development of mutual respect, open communication, and the potential for healing.
c. Interpret the patient's experience from a perspective that envisions possibilities, not limitations.
3. Advocacy and Empowering Patients and Families
a. Demonstrate a holistic approach to nursing practice committed to meeting the physical, psychological, social, and spiritual needs of the patient and family.
b. Facilitate patient/family decision making by assuring that adequate information is available.
c. Assist patient and family in the examination and clarification of their values within the context of the clinical situation.
d. Utilize creative approaches to empower patients and families, involving them in goal-setting, planning, and providing care.

Clinical Knowledge and Decision Making

1. Clinical Intuition/Forethought
a. Possess an intuitive grasp of the clinical situation by recognizing patterns and similarities in a problem without wasteful consideration of a large range of unfruitful possibilities.
b. Demonstrate exquisite foresight in anticipating problems and intervene before explicit diagnostic signs are evident.
2. Effective Management of Rapidly Changing Situations
a. Act decisively and delegate effectively in potentially life-threatening situations.
b. Communicate clearly and convincingly to make the clinical case in order to obtain timely and appropriate responses from physicians.
c. Maximize patient outcomes in situations that allow only short-term or indirect patient contact.

    d. Prioritize quickly in unpredictable situations and adjust strategies accordingly.

   3. Diagnostic Monitoring and Decision Making

    a. Selectively apply technology and correlate it to the patient's response.

    b. Critically evaluate own decision making and judgments.

Collaboration

   1. Personal Knowledge of Self

    a. Recognize knowledge of self to maintain objectivity and separate personal feelings within ethical/moral situations.

   2. Therapeutic Team

    a. Value the expertise of the team members and creatively coordinate resources to provide the highest quality care for patient/family.

    b. Influence practice by challenging the system and expanding boundaries to best meet the patient/family needs.

    c. Identify the dilemma and offer constructive coping strategies.

    d. Negotiate conflict by focusing on patient outcomes and promoting collaboration.

   3. Peer Support/Credibility

    a. Provide emotional and situational support for colleagues.

    b. Promote unit stability and encourage teamwork.

    c. Are sought out by colleagues for formal and informal consultation.

    d. Portray a professional image and positively influence practice.

FIRST COMMUNICATIONS WITH THE ENTIRE NURSING BODY

Following NPC approval, the workgroup presented the expert framework with distribution of supporting narratives to the Resource Group for their dissemination. The Narrative Workgroup also made a presentation to the nurses at large at their quarterly assembly to increase awareness, elicit feedback, and harness understanding and support. The response from staff and nursing leadership was overwhelmingly positive. It was with great pride that our learnings from the narratives were shared. Numerous people commented in amazement on how the framework captured many aspects of the practice that were not readily apparent before. The level of complexity of care and attention to care of the entire family was particularly striking.

NEXT STEPS

The workgroup developed the other frameworks of Novice, Advanced Beginner, Competent, and Proficient by using a similar process, that is, create the framework, test it, ensure its approval, and distribute it to others. Definitions for each of the five stages were grounded in the original work from the Dreyfus Model of Skill Acquisition (Exhibit 3–4). The themes of Caring, Clinical Knowledge and Decision Making, and Collaboration served as the template through each of all the developmental stages (Exhibit 3–5). A complete description of each framework is included in Appendix C.

VALIDATION

The members used an external validation process to ensure that the descriptive statements in the framework were grounded in the narratives of the SLMC nurses rather than in our ideal or imagined state. Benner Associates and the Director of Nursing Education for Aurora HealthCare provided the validation for each framework, using its supporting narrative base.

CREATING AN UNDERSTANDING OF THE NEW MODEL

Creating opportunities for learning about the model and the ways in which the narratives truly defined the practice was a sizable undertaking. It was necessary to create dialogue and understanding of how narratives illustrated the stages of skill development for caring, clinical knowledge and decision making, and collaboration. One successful strategy used to illustrate the changing perspectives of nurses along the developmental continuum involved stories about the care of the

Exhibit 3–4 Definitions of the Five Stages within the Clinical Practice Development Model

Stage	Definition
1 Novice	The Stage 1 novice nurse is a new graduate of a RN program and is in orientation. This nurse is obtaining knowledge and experience in clinical and technical skills. Under the guidance of a preceptor, the nurse collects objective data according to guidelines and rules obtained from nursing education and in orientation. The novice nurse utilizes this objective data and seeks assistance in making clinical decisions.
2 Advanced Beginner	Stage 2 advanced beginners are guided by policies and are most comfortable in a task environment. They describe a clinical situation from the viewpoint of what they need to do, rather than relating the context of the situation or how the patient responds. Advanced beginners practice from a theoretical knowledge base while they recognize and provide for routine patient needs.
3 Competent	Stage 3 competent nurses integrate theoretical knowledge with clinical experience in the care of patients and families. Care is delivered utilizing a deliberate, systematic approach and practice is guided by increasing awareness of patterns of patient responses in recurrent situations. The nurses demonstrate mastery of most technical skills, and begin to view clinical situations from a patient and family focus.
4 Proficient	Stage 4 nurses are proficient practitioners who have in-depth knowledge of nursing practice, perceive situations as a whole, and comprehend the significant elements based on previous experience. These nurses demonstrate the ability to recognize situational changes that require unplanned or unanticipated interventions. They

	respond to most situations with confidence, speed, and flexibility. Progression is from a task orientation to a holistic view of patient care. The nurses develop effective relationships with other caregivers and provide leadership within the health care team to formulate integrated approaches to care. They interpret the patient and family experiences from a perspective that begins to envision and create possibilities.
5 Expert	Stage 5 nurses are expert practitioners whose intuition and skill arise from comprehensive knowledge grounded in experience. Their practice is characterized by a flexible, innovative, and confident self-directed approach to patient and family care. Expert nurses operate from a deep understanding of the total situation. They put into perspective their own personal values and are able to encourage and support patient and family choices. Expert nurses collaborate with other caregivers to challenge and coordinate institutional resources to maximize advocacy for patient and family care in achieving the most effective outcomes.

Source: Courtesy of St. Luke's Medical Center, Milwaukee, Wisconsin.

Exhibit 3–5 St. Luke's Medical Center Clinical Practice Development Model: Excerpts

Stage I: Novice	Stage II: Advanced Beginner	Stage III: Competent	Stage IV: Proficient	Stage V: Expert
New graduate with little or no professional experience.	Utilizes theoretical knowledge (book knowledge)	Incorporates some experience. Sees limits of formal knowledge.	Integrates theoretical knowledge and experience.	Practices from extensive clinical experience.
Clinical Knowledge & Decision Making				
Learning P & P, Standards which will guide their practice.	Rule based. Uses P & P, Standards.	Completes Care Plans without help.	Consults with others when appropriate. Seeks out and/or provides assistance as needed.	Intuitive: zeroes in on problem without wasteful consideration of options.
Collects objective data, which can be recognized without situational experience.	Performs elemental analysis of information.	Limits the unexpected. Prefers status quo.	Still approaches new situations in analytical manner.	Synthesizes the parts into a whole.
Obtaining knowledge and experience in clinical and technical skills.	Sees isolated parts of the whole (what needs to be done).	Sets goals, plans and organizes consistently.	Sees changing relevance of situation. Recognizes patterns.	Sees the whole situation.
Requires guidance to identify the most relevant tasks to perform.	Functions best in task orientation.	Task mastery, provides standardized care.	Views situation more holistically. Envisions possibilities, not limitations.	Views situations holistically. Is flexible and innovative in approach.

Needs assistance with correlating theoretical knowledge to clinical situations.	Depends on others to respond to status changes they identify.	Responds in a conscious and deliberate manner to changing status.	Discriminates and responds to changing situation based on experience. Remains engaged with family.	Instinctively responds to rapidly changing situations.

Caring

Recognizes own feelings in patient/family relationships. Beginning to cope with reality of their own practice.	Maintains engagement with patient/family. Views situation in terms of what it demands of them. Validates practice through external sources.	Maintains involvement with family. Has sense of hyper-responsibility. Reflects on own impact re: patient outcome.	Establishes boundaries of therapeutic relationship-advocacy. Struggles with moral/ethical dilemmas.	Demonstrates strong presencing, understands meaning of health care changes for patient/family. Possesses knowledge of self and separates personal feelings from moral/ethical dilemmas.

Collaboration

Developing first professional relationships within the health care team.	Begins to see their own contribution to health care team.	Delegates to other members of health care team.	Mobilizes health care team. Persists in getting appropriate and timely responses.	Coordinates health care team for best patient/family outcome.

Source: Courtesy of St. Luke's Medical Center, Milwaukee, Wisconsin.

same patient from an expert and advanced beginner nurse. Both of the following stories illustrate excellence of practice within their stage of development. Notice the engagement and commitment to good practice that they both describe. New learners easily recognized the contrast between the two practitioners' stage of development.

Advanced Beginner Narrative from a Maternity Nurse. When I arrived at work for my P.M. shift, a group of nurses were discussing assignments for the evening. I overheard someone say, "Judy can handle that patient." I soon found out what my assignment would be that night. The patient I would be caring for had recently returned to our unit from an intensive care unit. She had become a "code" during recovery period following a cesarean delivery. Two feelings were going on inside me as I was getting the report from the day nurse. I felt afraid and excited by the challenge.

When I walked into her room for the first time, I was overwhelmed by the amount of tubes and machines. She had a foley, JVAC, an NG tube, and a peripheral IV. For an experienced nurse this might not seem intimidating, but I had only a year and a half in nursing. As I checked each tube and machine, I tried to talk to my patient and put her at ease. I found myself concentrating more on my assessment of the physical environment than on what she was saying.

My shift progressed and things improved. I was able to change my focus from the machines to the person connected to them. I was able to get to know her and learn about her experience. She shared her excitement about her new baby and her fears about her recovery. I felt it was a very rewarding day. I learned about the tubes and machines, but more importantly, about the person.

Courtesy of Judy Buskiewicz, RN

Expert Narrative from a Maternity Nurse. J. was a patient I cared for. She was a Gravida 1 Para 0 who had an emergency cesarean section for placenta previa and bleeding. Following her cesarean she was transferred to the Medical Respiratory Intensive Care Unit following a silent code on our unit. I cared for J. following her return to OB.

J. didn't look up as I entered the room. When I spoke she diverted her gaze. Responses were very limited. This patient was described to me in report as scared and at times demanding. The focus was on her many physician needs (assessments, vitals, drain, NG) and on meeting those needs.

Meeting J. briefly to say good morning, as I often do with most patients, gave me some thoughts on how to work with her, not to her. Sure, she had many physical cares that had to be tended to, but what about those emotional needs that hadn't been addressed?

I sat on her bed, I searched out her eyes, we made contact; and together we planned her morning. I stayed with her as she provided care for her new baby. At times we would talk, but at other times silence seemed most comfortable. Finally, she could open up. I listened and explored her experience with birth, near death, and slow recovery. She had not spoken of any of her birth events previously. She shared her fears; she tried to piece together her experiences over the previous two weeks. I listened to her. I reached out and hugged her and cried with her as she described her thoughts of knowing she was dying and would not be here for her new baby.

I wanted to help her through her own experience. Her storytelling was piecing her puzzle together. She needed mothering more than she needed my focus on her physical care. She needed my mothering, my true caring and concern, my confidence in her ability to heal physically and emotionally. She needed my reaching out so she could reach out and mother herself and her baby. Sitting with her, touching, sharing, explaining her physical concerns to her, exploring her concerns, helped give her what she needed to heal. Energy level improved, appetite increased, diarrhea decreased. She spoke of how good she felt. She wanted to keep her baby with her.

Surely I provided the physical care she needed, but I also provided an opportunity for her to incorporate her birth and near death experience into herself. Her energy, now increasing, allowed for more activity with her baby and family. I could step away and become the onlooker as she assumed more responsibility. That feeling of knowing what to focus on so this patient could make sense of her experience and continue in her transition to motherhood was priority for my care.

Courtesy of Katherine Kuchan, RN

Exhibit 3–6 displays the changing perspectives of nurses along the developmental continuum in the Caring Domain, along with excerpts from the previous two stories.

Exhibit 3–7 shows how descriptive statements embedded in an actual narrative correlate with the CPDM framework's practice themes and characteristics. This is another strategy the team used to help learners understand and appreciate the way in which narratives defined the practice and how the framework was evident in the narratives.

Exhibit 3–6 Changing Perspectives Along the Continuum. Domain: Caring

Novice	Advanced Beginner	Competent	Proficient	Expert
• Responds to comfort needs • Recognizes own feelings in pt/family relationships	• Approaches pts and families with compassion • Provide comfort to patients • Recognize importance of therapeutic relationships	• Individualize care and begin to recognize personhood of pt and family • Learning to establish and practice within the boundaries of therapeutic relationships	• Establish trusting therapeutic relationships through understanding of specific and relevant aspects of the pt/family experiences • Realize the significant impact that life events and health status changes have—offer guidance & support • Recognize that healing requires more than physical interventions, promote environment grounded in empathy, kindness, and deep regard for the individual	• "Being with" vs. "doing to" a patient • Demonstrate a deep understanding of the unique meaning of health, illness, and disease on pt/family • Actively listen in an effort to understand, though not necessary agree with pt/family choices • Promote healing by helping the pt cope with the fears and concerns with life changes • Provide environment of hope and trust with mutual respect and open communication • Utilize creative approaches to empower patients and families, involving them in goal-setting, planning and providing care

Mrs. O. was a 34-yr.-old woman who, immediately after childbirth, suffered a life threatening hemorrhage. She spent two days in ICU and was not returning to the OB floor.

Advanced Beginner Caring for Mrs. O.

When I walked into her room for the first time, I was overwhelmed by the amount of tubes and machines. She had a foley, IVAC, NG tube, and IV. As I checked each tube and machine, I tried to talk to my patient and put her at ease. I found myself concentrating more on my assessment on the physical environment than on what she was saying.

My shift progressed and things improved. I was able to change my focus from machines to the person connected to them. I was able to know her and learn about her experience. She shared her excitement about her new baby and her fears about her recovery. . . . Judy Buskiewicz, RN

Expert Caring for Mrs. O.

I sat on her bed, I searched out her eyes, we made contact and together we planned her morning. . . . At times we would talk but at other times silence seemed most comfortable. Finally she could open up. I listened and explored her experience with birth, near death, and slow recovery. She shared her fears. . . . I wanted to help her through her own experience. Her story-telling was piecing her puzzle together. She needed mothering, my true caring and concern, my confidence in her ability to heal physically and emotionally. She needed my reaching out so she could reach out and mother herself and her baby. . . . Energy level improved, appetite increased, diarrhea decreased. She spoke of how good she felt. She wanted to keep her baby with her. I could step away and become the onlooker as she assumed more responsbility. That feeling of knowing what to focus on so this patient could make sense of her experience and continue in her transition to motherhood was priority for my care. . . . Katherine Kuchan, RN

Source: Courtesy of St. Luke's Medical Center, Milwaukee, Wisconsin.

Exhibit 3-7 Expert characteristics of practice revealed in excerpts of a narrative.

... After getting report from the noc shift nurse, I made rounds of the unit to further assess the patients who sounded extremely critical in report and to confirm the few potential transfers. At about 0900 the patient Mr. Z. was sent back to surgery on nocs for bleeding had returned to the unit with the anesthesiologist at the bedside. The patient's VSS was a bit hypertensive so the primary nurse started nipride per standing order; however after just a few ccs there was a drastic drop in BP. The nipride was DC'd. Positioned at the head of the bed, I put the patient in Trendelenburg ... we all watched the monitor waiting for the MAP to go above the 60 mmHg required for adequate brain perfusion ... hoping the hypotension was drug induced. Minutes passed showing little improvement. Without comment I opened the IVs wide, the anesthesiologist bolused neosynephrine and *I paged the surgeon* (**thinking to myself this poor patient's bleeding internally** *and his surgeon has been up all night with him struggling to save his life*).

Now at the bedside and after hearing report of what had occurred, the surgeon stated he felt the hypotension was nipride induced. STAT labs came back - the Hct was 23 but comparable to prior values - ABGs WNL, no drainage from the chest tubes. I suggested a CXR to the surgeon and he nodded. *I called the order to the secretary.* (thinking to myself; 20 minutes had passed since admission... was there adequate vital organ perfusion **...if he survived, what would be his brain function, quality of life** ...he's got to get back to surgery STAT!). I asked the surgeon if I should alert OR for the patient's return and he said "pack him up I'm taking him back. Oh! I'd just told his wife he was OK."

OR was called and I returned to the bedside and assisted the primary nurse in transporting the patient. The surgeon came to us and asked if we agreed the hypotension was drug induced. M. (the nurse) said "I disagree." and I said "I think he's got a chest full of blood, probably blew another graft." **My next thoughts were for the family. We've got to tell his poor wife.** M. said "I'll go talk to her. She knows me from our brief talk this morning."

When Mr. Z. finally returned to the unit - 2 nurses at the bedside ready to admit. *Again I observed from the bedside, available to assist if needed. M. asked me to call blood bank and inform them that the patient would now be on a FFP IV drip (1 unit every 2 hours). I requested they bring*

Source: Courtesy of St. Luke's Medical Center, Milwaukee, Wisconsin.

continues

up each unit without further calls and promised to inform them if the order was DC'd. The admission went like clock work - nipride and arfonad required to keep SBP less than 110; NSR, labs pending, moderate to large CT drainage, Baer hugger on, CI almost 2.

I called Mr. Z's family up for their visit. At last his poor wife and son could see him, talk to him, hold his hand, I knew they'd been riding a frightening roller coaster for almost 24 hours. They were exhausted emotionally and physically - weren't fully comprehending as the surgeon explained that a graft from the aorta had broken loose ..

Mary Ihde, RN

EXPERT: These are selected characteristics of practice from the expert stage of CPDM.

Domain: CARING

- **establish trusting relationship with patient/family grounded in "being with" not "doing to" a patient.**
- **demonstrate deep understanding of unique meaning of health, illness and disease on pt/family.**
- **provide a healing environment of hope and trust.**

Domain: Clinical Knowledge/Decision Making

- possess an intuitive grasp of the clinical situation by recognizing patterns and similarities in problem without wasteful consideration of unfruitful possibilities.
- demonstrate exquisite foresight in anticipating problems and intervene before explicit diagnostic signs are evident
- communicate clearly and convincingly to make the clinical case in order to obtain timely and appropriate responses from physicians
- prioritize quickly in unpredictable situations and adjust strategies accordingly
- selectively applies technology and correlate to patient's response

Domain: COLLABORATION

- *Value the expertise of the team members and creatively coordinate resources*
- *provide emotional and situational support for colleagues*
- *promote unit stability and encourage teamwork*

PROMOTING LEADERSHIP PROFICIENCY

The team used strategies that strengthened the competency of the staff leadership, CNSs, and managers to operate in the new model. They did this through educational sessions; small group dialogue sessions identifying characteristics of practice and staging actual narratives; and providing written validation packages. Although all agreed that the novice to expert model made a lot of sense and they could recall their own experiences at different developmental stages throughout the years, we found everyone needed to invest some time in acquiring the skills for working with the new model. This investment ranged from a few hours to many hours and several attempts at validation for some.

IMPLEMENTATION

A Steering Committee of key stakeholders in the organization guided the implementation process for the CPDM. Its formation occurred at the same time as the Narrative Workgroup began its work. The processes used to guide the implementation were complex and each governance council's accountabilities were realized. The details of the work of the Steering Committee are described in the next chapter (Chapter 4).

Chapter 4

Use of a Steering Committee to Guide Implementation

Julie Raaum, Nora Ladewig, and Barbara Haag-Heitman

Never doubt that a small group of thoughtful,
committed citizens can change the world.
Indeed, it is the only thing that ever has.
—Margaret Mead

A steering committee was formed to guide implementation of our Clinical Practice Development Model (CPDM) due to the magnitude and complexity of this change. Indeed, this new practice model would have impact beyond its individual effect on our 700 nurses. Other parts of the system such as orientation and practice expectations, as well as wage and salary, would be influenced. The CPDM implementation was the first major project undertaken in the new shared governance structure that demanded considerable coordination and system linkage with other parts of the organization. The Steering Committee membership consisted of the chairs of the shared governance councils; the Professional Nursing Assembly (PNA) President and the President-Elect, the Vice President of Nursing, the Director of Nursing Operations, the Recruitment and Retention Specialist, the Vice President of Human Resources, the Director of Corporate Nursing Education, and the chairperson of the narrative workgroup commissioned by the Practice council. This group of 13 people was

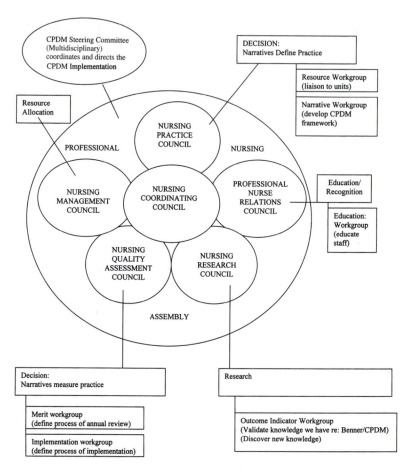

Figure 4.1 Council and Committee Accountabilities for CPDM

Source: Courtesy of St. Luke's Medical Center, Milwaukee, Wisconsin.

accountable to move the project along and to anticipate the resources and connections that the councils needed so that their decisional work could move forward. This collaborative effort facilitated a whole systems perspective for the project and, in particular, gave direction to the council chairpersons. Consequently each leader could formulate proactive agendas for their respective councils that would guide and direct their work and decision making in a time-efficient manner, in accordance with the project timeline. Figure 4–1 illustrates the relationship of the Steering Committee to the Shared Governance Councils, along with their specific accountabilities related to the CPDM.

The following account describes the perspective of the Vice President of Human Resources and the Recruitment/Retention Specialist as stakeholders on the Steering Committee.

> There were five areas that I was mainly concerned about from a Human Resource point of view. It was important that the Clinical Practice Development Model promote a positive employee atmosphere and be able to offer us a sound competitive advantage in the market place. Alignment with the overall goals and objectives of the organization and support from the physicians were also significant factors. Additionally, the ability to effectively and efficiently administer the program was essential.
>
> Courtesy of Frank Cummins
> Vice President of Human Resources
> St. Luke's Medical Center

The project timeline specified a 13-month implementation period following the approval of the entire CPDM by the Nursing Practice Council. During this time, education about the model continued through the Professional Relations Councils, and the peer review process was designed by the Nursing Quality Council. Much of the Management Council's focus was on resource allocation to support the development of expertise in nursing practice via the implementation of the CPDM. A full description of the management considerations is found in Chapter 8. The Nursing Research council began to explore outcome measures and their work is detailed in Chapter 7. All councils worked closely together to assure a smooth transition. One of the goals of the Steering Committee was to complete the entire transition by the common salary review date in spring. Another factor that influenced the time line involved a research study, designed to investigate a salaried model of compensation for nurses. In order for data collection to begin for this project, common salaries and job descriptions needed to be identified and in place. A somewhat compressed timeline was the result of these two factors.

The work of the Steering Committee was communicated to the rest of the nursing staff through a number of avenues. The most successful vehicle for broad-based communication was the house-wide nursing newsletter, the *Interchange*, which was already in place and published monthly. Reports from the Steering Committee about the progress of the nursing councils in redesigning the clinical advancement program were published in each issue. Since all members of the Nursing Coordinating council were also Steering Committee members, the shared governance system had information dispersed among councils and workgroups easily.

DECISION TO USE NARRATIVES TO MEASURE PRACTICE

With the development of the CPDM complete, the major contribution from the Nursing Practice Council was finished. The next phase of the process involved creating a mechanism to evaluate and measure practice, which would be the work of the Nursing Quality Assessment Council (NQAC).

Having closely followed the work of the Nursing Practice Council, the NQAC had grown in their understanding of how clinical narratives could define practice. It became evident that narrative accounts could be used to measure bedside practice and this methodology quickly became central in the redesign of the clinical advancement program. The decision to use narratives to determine a nurse's place on the developmental continuum of clinical practice was the springboard for future paradigm shifts in the St. Luke's nursing culture and behaviors.

Publicizing the decision to use narratives to define and measure nursing practice increased the nurses' awareness of the decisional process of the house-wide shared governance councils. This decision had the potential to impact every nurse in the institution, and despite the many attempts to share the development of the model, many nurses were still not aware that they would be evaluated based on their own account of their practice. Doubts and concerns were expressed by nurses who had not kept themselves abreast with the developments as to who had made these decisions and what was their authority. The new need-to-know created a period of great learning for the nursing division.

The authority commensurate with the accountabilities vested in the governance councils was beginning to be understood by the staff as the implementation process rolled out. In the past, decisions of this nature and magnitude had always resided with the chief nurse executive (CNE). Indeed we were discovering that this was the beginning of a very different and positive way of doing nursing business.

The constant flow of inquiries and responses about the CPDM from our colleagues made it a very taxing time to be a staff nurse in a leadership role on the nursing governance councils. But it was clear to us that the supportive foundation for change had been well constructed and carefully laid over the past year. It was challenging helping our peers grow in their understanding and acceptance of the novice to expert developmental framework while we were learning our new roles of staff nurse leadership. Staff participating on the shared governance councils were learning a new role—that of change agent. The staff's vulnerabilities and anxieties needed to be addressed and transformed into positive energy to keep the implementation of CPDM moving in the right direction. Helping staff work through the uncertain stages in this change process was an essential form of our change agent role.

SEPARATING CLINICAL ADVANCEMENT FROM ANNUAL REVIEW

Using narrative accounts of practice to describe and evaluate nursing practice along a developmental continuum was central to the redesign of the nursing recognition and advancement system. One of the most significant and visible decisions that resulted was to separate the annual performance review process from the peer review process for clinical promotion and advancement.

Through the work of the NQAC, the content of the annual performance review was redefined. Common organizational behaviors for the review were refocused on more citizenship behaviors as identified in the employee handbook. These criteria were as basic as attendance and service management expectations. In addition, common components generic to all staff, such as adherence to the nursing standards and competencies, were more clearly defined. As the merit review process is a function of the Annual Performance Review, it remained the accountability of the unit-based mangers. This left the opportunity for true peer review of nursing practice to reveal itself in the process designed for clinical excellence to be recognized and rewarded using the CPDM. The peer review process is more fully discussed in Chapter 5.

The separation of advancement from merit afforded us opportunity to create a clear focus on clinical excellence in an environment based on peer trust and respect. Since narratives are first-person accounts of actual events, the writers often reveal more than they may intend. A climate of trust and respect is required to ensure that the narratives are read in their own terms, that assumptions on the part of the readers will be clarified, and that any questions will be raised with the writer. This new position and intent demands its own process and time allotment, supporting its separation from the annual review.

CPDM IMPLEMENTATION WORKGROUP

The NQAC details on how narratives would be used to place and advance nurses along the developmental continuum of the CPDM was the work of the NQAC. Another workgroup was commissioned from this council and was charged with making specific recommendations about the number of narratives used, and with drafting a policy of implementation of CPDM. This workgroup would report their findings to the Quality Council for final prioritization and decision making.

Specific criteria were used for selection of the workgroup membership. A member of the NQAC would lead the group to assure clear direction for the work and linkage to the decision-making body. To sustain the momentum and build on the foundational decisions made up to this time, representation from two previous workgroups, the Narrative Workgroup, out of the Nursing Practice Council, and the Annual Performance Workgroup, out of the NQAC, were recruited. Additional staff nurse representation was solicited through the monthly newsletter, the *Interchange*, to assure a broad representation. Because of the nature of the work, staff made up the majority of the workgroup membership. There was a tremendous response. It seemed that everyone was interested in shaping the evaluation process for one reason or another. The workgroup membership was closed at 27 members. This was a much larger group than originally imagined; however, after lengthy discussions at the council level it was determined that this composition would be the most representative and essential for facilitating a smooth and successful implementation and transition to the CPDM. The wisdom of this decision became evident as the process moved forward.

During the formation of this group it became clear that a wide range of understanding of the CPDM existed. It was evident early on that this group could not meet the tasks it was commissioned to accomplish without first doing some foundational work with the membership. The core of this work was modeled after the lessons learned in the development of the narrative workgroup out of the Practice Council. To assist the membership with their knowledge of the CPDM, and engage them in the methodology, it was decided to have them write their own narratives and identify characteristics of practice from the CPDM. Those members who were prior narrative group members assisted them in this process. Members' narratives were then shared in the workgroup and they grew together in their understanding and trust of the CPDM. Through the process they discovered how the clinical accountings from the narratives could be discussed in terms of the characteristics of practice and common themes as outlined in the CPDM.

This strategy was very successful in helping the workgroup membership, who were in a key decisional position, appreciate the correlation between experiencing the model and understanding the model. As a result of this learning, the workgroup realized that for staff nurses to truly understand the CPDM they should experience it through the writing of their own narratives, aided by reflection and conversations with others who could assist them in reading the practice characteristics. This strategic group had unmistakably experienced the power and wisdom imbedded in the narratives. They also now recognized how clinical narratives reveal the skill and practical knowledge embedded in practice that could not be measured in the old career ladder. This paradigm shift guided the workgroup in its recommendation that all staff would participate in the writing of narratives and the use of a peer review process to review them using the CPDM framework. The result would be the recognition that would result in their placement on the five-stage developmental continuum. This process would be called "transition" and was to be completed in the time specified by the Steering Committee. Additionally, the workgroup recommended that no nurse would be grandfathered into the new model and no nurse would be placed on the continuum without developing narratives and participating in the peer review process. The NQAC adopted these two strategic recommendations.

LEARNING ABOUT THE CONCERNS OF STAFF

In keeping with our learning that true understanding of the new model occurred by experiencing it through the narratives, we recognized the next challenge was to reach yet more staff. Knowing the concerns of each nurse on this workgroup, it stood to reason that nurses across the nursing organization had fears, concerns, and questions that needed a forum for expression. This understanding resulted in an increased effort to communicate with those groups of nurses not directly involved with the transition to the new model. A month-long focused effort was targeted to discuss concerns, address rumors, identify additional educational needs related to the CPDM, and develop narratives. Unit leadership was asked to dedicate a portion of their monthly staff meetings specific to the CPDM. Throughout this time the Implementation Workgroup members communicated with unit leadership to obtain their feedback on issues that needed to be addressed to further support implementation. Areas of particular concern centered around understanding the validity of using narratives and the peer review process for determining placement on the novice to expert continuum. Personal vulnerabilities and concerns about trust and confidentiality also surfaced. Some staff wanted to know about the plans for quality control, including an appeal process. Other questions were raised around equity and subjectivity, validity and reliability of the model. Chapter 12 more fully discusses these concepts. These issues, along with the concerns voiced regarding pay, were compiled. Issues not specific to the process of implementation were passed up to the chair of the Nursing Quality Assessment Council for discussion at the Nursing Coordinating Council and the Steering Committee. This facilitated the linkage of these issues with the council(s) accountable for that work.

Concurrently, the workgroup was learning from other organizations, which had used the novice to expert framework for the basis of promotion, about their experiences and process. Several of the institutions contacted had also worked with Benner Associates. Telephone inquiry was made by a member of the workgroup using a guided telephone interview tool. Topics included the model of nursing leadership currently in place, size of nursing staff, use of novice to expert model, mechanism(s) for merit and promotion, portfolio components for annual review, and use of clinical narratives. We found that all organizations were large hospitals or medical centers with some form of shared leadership, all had some portfolio component for annual review, none had separated merit from promotion, and none had used narratives exclusively for the basis of promotion. This information helped stimulate and clarify our own thinking. It became evident that we were unique in our approach about the sole use of narratives for advancement and the separation of advancement from annual performance review.

DEVELOPING NEW UNDERSTANDING

Out of the team learning experiences done by the Implementation Workgroup around the CPDM grew an appreciation for the similarity versus the diversity of its membership. Dialogue began to shift focus from what was done differently on each unit to acknowledging the shared experiences of nursing along the continuum of patient care across the organization. The language of the CPDM had shifted our perspective to the whole, and unified the workgroup membership. For the first time, we clearly recognized the barriers that had become part of our practice culture, such as the perceived ICU elitism and segregation of units based on their specialty care. It was freeing to be released from old ways of interpreting our work and our coworkers.

This new understanding was shared beyond the workgroup members, as they opened up new dialogue on their units about the benefits of the CPDM and the new peer review process. An increasing number of nurses grew in their awareness and comprehension of the changes as the 27 workgroup members carried the message back to their different areas of the hospital. These members created a ripple effect of shared vision across the organization. This workgroup became the opinion leaders who created areas of support for the model among the remainder of the nursing staff.

As a result of this new perspective, it became the recommendation that sharing practice through peer review be done at the house-wide versus unit level as part of the transition process. Although this was considered ideal for nurses at all stages, because of the large volume of nurses in the organization, the NQAC decided to make application and panel review at the house-wide level for Stage 4 (Proficient) and Stage 5 (Expert) applicants. We were excited about the opportunity to acknowledge heterogeneity in our nursing practice through house-wide peer review, which could be very powerful in creating a shared understanding of the practice. The house-wide peer review also appealed to those concerned with the integrity and validity of the process should each unit manage it. Placing nurses on the developmental continuum through a house-wide mechanism was clearly a tremendous human and fiscal resource expenditure. It was a very visible sign to the staff of the administrative support for the CPDM. It was consideration of the tremendous number of staff that would need to transition that led the NQAC to decide to make application and panel review for Stage 2 (Advanced Beginner) and Stage 3 (Competent) part of the work of unit-based quality councils. The units were directed to mimic a process consistent with the house-wide peer review process. This decision afforded yet another opportunity for more staff involvement in the process.

Further consultation with Benner Associates was arranged for the Implementation Workgroup. The issues generated from those focused unit-level discussions helped set the framework for the consultation. The majority of considerations centered on the use of narratives. Issues of subjectivity, fabrication, and poor writing skills made for weighty discussion. Through our consultative learning, we developed more skill and confidence in the methodology and recognized that these issues were not sound. As a result, the workgroup recommended that to accomplish the transition from the old career ladder levels to the developmental stages identified in CPDM, each staff nurse would write and submit three narratives to a peer review panel.

While the large numbers in this workgroup were often a barrier to efficient decision making, the size allowed for the creation of subgroups within the membership to accomplish a large volume of work in a short period of time. With agendas tightly set and a timeline to direct the focus, this workgroup accomplished its objective in five months. Their recommendations for the final implementation policy were adopted by the NQAC. The result of intense effort with and within this workgroup helped the members become the critical mass that successfully implemented CPDM within our institution. We had found the "opinion leaders" described by Wilson and were moving toward an early majority of nurses committed to the new structure.

CHAMPIONS FOR CHANGE

To successfully accomplish the transition collaboration and partnership among the staff and leadership was imperative. The unit-based managers and Clinical Nurse Specialists (CNSs) provided the necessary support and guidance needed for successful implementation. They too were learning the model at the same time and experienced similar vulnerabilities as the staff. Their ability to openly support the evolving process helped the staff leadership be more confident, flexible, and creative in their own processes. By communicating their belief in the validity and credibility of the new model, the implementation process was much less difficult for all staff.

The CNS group became champions of the model as they recognized the great potential for impacting on staff development and clinical excellence. Several CNSs had been key contributors to the model development and were skilled at communicating the strengths of the new system to their colleagues. Their largest contribution came from their commitment to coaching the nursing staff through the process. They became the primary coaching group as this skill was already inherent in the role and part of their practice accountabilities. The value of staff having the support of a coach was recognized early in the implementation and has remained a powerful tool for success in the ongoing maintenance and growth of the model. The coaching role is fully explored in Chapter 6.

During this change period, as is typical, there was some resistance and testing of the decisions made; some nurses strongly opposed the model, while others questioned whether the transition would really happen. Some tested the authority of the new governance model by trying old ways of bringing about change, such as complaining to nursing administration, other administrators, and even physicians. These efforts were not successful and added to the collective learning about the new way of doing business. The nursing leadership group recognized these efforts on the part of the staff as typical reactions to change and felt secure in knowing that they had full administrative support for implementing the model. This tension brought about by the change created a new demand for clear and continuous communication with the staff.

MODEL EDUCATION

Once the transition criteria and process were clearly defined by the NQAC, it was time for the Professional Nursing Relations Council (PNRC) to take action. It was their charge to communicate information and educate the nursing staff about the model and its implementation. Members of this council were creative in their approach and employed a number of different options for providing education and information to nursing staff members at varying levels of understanding.

Because the house-wide newsletter, the *Interchange,* was already in place and had been given the position of communication vehicle for shared governance activities, it was used as the principle means of communicating to all staff. In addition to the regular columns about the Steering Committee work, reports from other CPDM workgroups were included and a "question-and-answer" section was added to help with sharing information. To further communicate the decision-making accountability of the councils regarding CPDM and other topics, a "Decision Page" was added that summarized council decisions from meetings held during the time period between publications. This method of communicating decisions helped the staff to identify what they had to know about CPDM as well as other issues and to determine which council was accountable for a particular decision. Several narratives from the staff like the one that follows were published in the *Interchange* to help educate the staff with narrative writing.

> J.R. was a heart transplant patient who was post-op day three. He had been progressing fairly well in spite of the fact that he waited for months in the hospital for his transplant. The nurse who gave me

report that day said he was a difficult patient and wouldn't make any effort to do any of his activities. She had requested a change in assignment for the next day.

From my experience with 'difficult' patients, I find that the best way to take care of them is to allow them to have some control over their environment. Their anxiety often stems from feeling a loss of control. They don't like being dependent on others for help if they are used to being independent. I decided to go into my patient's room without any preconceived notions about him in spite of what the nurse had told me.

That day, I gave J.R. the nursing care he needed, but I let him make some decisions about how he would like to do things and was very flexible to meet his needs. I sat by his bedside and talked with him about his condition and treatment plan. I encouraged him to tell me what he was feeling. I felt that in a short time I was able to earn his trust. His kids came to visit him that day for the first time since his transplant. Although it went against visiting policy, I felt that it was important for them to visit for J.R.'s sake as well as the kids', so I let them come in. This was questioned by the staff but I defended myself by saying that it was for the benefit of the patient. The patient was in a closed room and the children were not disturbing any of the other patients.

At the end of the day, J.R. told me that he did not get along with the nurse on the previous shift. He said that he realized the importance of activity and was willing to do it, but she did not give him time to do the activities at his own pace. I did not defend her or share in his criticism, as I was not there to see his encounters with her, but I merely listened. He had done a good job of participating in his activities that day for me and I saw a lot of progress. I told him this and encouraged him to keep up the good work.

When I gave shift report to the next nurse, I explained to her that J.R. needed to do things at his own pace and she would have better participation from him if she allowed him to participate in his care decisions. I also made a care plan that specified ways to let J.R. have some control over his own care.

Courtesy of Karen Gustrau, RN, CVICU, Stage 5

Many units at St. Luke's Medical Center had an already established unit-based newsletter as an additional form of information sharing, and these newsletters were also used to communicate the latest updates regarding CPDM implementation. This format was used to give staff specifics about such items as their unit-based councils and timelines for submitting narratives. Units also published narratives from among their staff via this mechanism.

Every opportunity to present and discuss the CPDM was seized. The Professional Nursing Assembly (PNA) meetings, which are the business meetings of the shared governance councils, were held regularly and featured updates about the model and implementation at each meeting. The members of the Steering Committee also volunteered to attend unit staff meetings to provide information about the model and answer questions staff had about the process. Several units used this mechanism to help communicate the process. In addition, the Professional Nursing Relations Council held several open forums to help answer questions and listen to the concerns of the staff. Attendance at these forums was often large and often was a mixed audience of information-seekers along with some nonsupporters. Whenever Benner Associates were present for consultation, they met with staff during special open forums to assisting in understanding the use of narratives to capture clinical reasoning across time and to make the often invisible caring work of nurses visible. This was well received by the staff. The session that Patricia Benner attended was particularly memorable to the staff. She read their narratives during the forum and publicly acknowledged the practice. Staff who attended spoke of how good it felt to be part of that experience and how they furthered their understanding about how narratives could define the practice.

Over time, these exchanges continued to expose the nursing staff to new learnings and dialogue with their peers. This was yet another marker of the subtle culture change occurring organizationally in nursing. It was the staff, in their new leadership roles, that facilitated much of the discussion and conflict resolution that had been done by the managers and CNSs in the past governance model.

Additional opportunities to learn about the CPDM along with a class on how to actually write a narrative were created.

Resource binders were created for distribution to every nursing unit. They contained several educational pieces in addition to sample narratives. Information about CPDM and what nurses needed to know to navigate the process of peer review were also included, along with a reference list of the names of all nurses who had participated in the development and implementation process, and a brief overview of accountabilities related to CPDM. Journal articles written by the Benners were placed in packets. These resource binders remain an integral part of the unit-based strategy to support staff through the preparation for the peer review process.

TRANSITION CELEBRATION

The PNRC was also responsible for the celebrations that occurred on many levels during and after the transition to CPDM. When the paneling process was initiated, the PNRC sponsored a large kickoff event that was held on all three shifts. This event featured an "ice cream social" theme where staff were encouraged to make their own ice cream sundaes and tour poster displays depicting the CPDM process. The names and pictures of the nurses involved in the development of the model and the transition efforts were also showcased. In addition, the introduction of the CPDM to others outside nursing was done through the distribution in the cafeteria of the following one-page narrative titled "A Story of Nursing Practice."

> One afternoon while I was sitting at the desk charting on a patient I noticed quite a bit of commotion coming from one of our rooms. I knew that a man in his 'thirties had come in within the hour with chest pain. I could tell from the number of staff in his room that he was probably having a myocardial infarction (MI) and could sense that the level of anxiety in the room was high. I saw the patient writhing on the cart, presumably in pain, and several nurses, a physician and resident, an EKG tech, all in his room. The monitor alarms were singing, voices were loud and staccato. The patient was moaning and just couldn't rest still.
> I went into the room to see how I could help. I could see on his monitor that he was having frequent PVCs and runs of V tach and

that he was getting lidocaine to treat it, but it didn't seem to be working. He had received morphine for his pain. It also didn't seem to be working. People kept yelling at him to lie still. (It's funny how we seem to think anxious patients are hearing impaired!)

Instinctively, I stepped to his bedside, near his head. I noticed that his eyes were closed, that he was grimacing in pain and moving about on the bed. I touched his shoulder, called his name and asked him to open his eyes and look at me. He did. Clearly he was terrified. I told him my name and that I was just going to be there for him while the others were working to help him. I began by acknowledging how frightening this must be for him. I wanted to alter his perception of what must have seemed to be an overwhelmingly threatening, chaotic situation, to a helpful, controlled one. So I began by sorting out for him all the different sensations coming at him at once. I told him that while he was having a heart attack, that he was at a hospital that specialized in taking care of this, that he was in excellent hands and that the staff was working very hard to give him the very best treatment. I told him that for the time being, all he had to attend to was my voice, that if he chose to keep his eyes closed I would let him know what was happening. I also suggested to him that while the staff was working, that there were things that he could do to help himself, like his breathing. I asked him to take a deep breath and feel his chest and shoulder muscles loosen. I explained that his heart was hurting because it needed more oxygen and told him how to breathe to bring more oxygen to his heart. I suggested that maybe he could even picture how the blood vessels around his heart were able to open up and carry all this oxygen to his heart. Then I told him that sometimes when there is a heart attack, that the heart wanted to skip beats but that he was being given medication to help his heart beat regularly. I suggested that he might even be beginning to feel that medication working already to provide a steady, regular rhythm.

Within moments, he appeared to relax, he stopped grimacing and writhing in pain, and his heart rhythm became regular. The entire anxiety level in the room decreased. The physician, who was standing at the bedside, looked up and said, 'Wow, how did you do that?'

The entire intervention took minutes.

Staff Nurse, Emergency Services

The skillful integration of the nurse's caring practices with her expert clinical knowledge and decision-making skills and teamwork were readily apparent in this example. Those outside nursing easily acknowledged her exquisite practice and began to appreciate how much one could tell from just one story. The introduction of the CPDM was also announced via tent cards on the cafeteria tables. Special buttons that acknowledged the applicant's completion of the process were given to the applicants by the peer review panel to celebrate the applicant's achievement and to stimulate additional dialogue about the process. At large staff who were not yet staged often approached those with buttons to gain further understanding about the process. Each unit was encouraged to develop its own celebration format, and several created unique ways to recognize staff for successfully completing the process. The unit manager and CNS usually arranged the recognition mechanisms, which ranged from flowers for the applicants on the day of their review to lunches to honor people who were staged. The meaning of this celebration is described by one of the staff: "I got recognition from my manager and CNS...the pin, the letter, and I think we had a lunch too. That was very nice."

The need for recognition and celebration of the paneling process and movement to the CPDM model varied widely among staff. For this reason, units were not given distinct directions regarding celebration and recognition events, but rather were encouraged to design such events in a manner that would be acceptable to all.

COMPLETION OF TRANSITION

Once the paneling process started, there was additional momentum and support for the CPDM. Many staff stepped forward early and expressed support and satisfaction with the new system. Others adopted a "wait-and-see" attitude, letting their peers go through the process first and then learning from the experience prior to jumping in. Still, some staff nurses who had hoped that the entire process would fade away or be driven away now were planning their response to the expectation of participation. It was clearly expected that all nurses in the staff position would make the transition from the old career ladder model of evaluation to the new CPDM. The transition period was a time of great learning about the strengths of our practice as well as factors that were impeding it. The Management and Steering Committee (see Chapter 8) addressed institutional impediments. New and lasting positive relationships were formed between the staff and leadership. These factors helped focus our resources, strengthen our collective practice, celebrate the true essence of nursing.

The secretarial staff was instrumental in the success of the transition. Their coordination helped the process go smoothly despite the obstacles. There were several logistical difficulties stemming from the need to schedule many meeting rooms for over 700 panels to take place, which they creatively overcame. Staff was guaranteed privacy for the review process and the applicant interview, which meant that only one panel could be housed in a room, regardless of size. We were also challenged by the demand for qualified panel members. Calls for panel members were made throughout the process, and for the transition, managers and CNSs not coaching the applicant also served as panel members. After transition, the decision was made to limit panel membership to staff nurses only. (See peer review, Chapter 5, for more detail about panel member training and peer review process.)

The transition process was accomplished by the deadline through the dedication and commitment of many nurses. However, the fundamental paradigm shifting experienced by the nursing organization has extended well beyond the transition period.

EVALUATING THE PROCESS

The Nursing Research Council commissioned a workgroup to learn more about how to support nurses undergoing tremendous organizational changes. This workgroup specifically focused on nurses' attitudes and perceptions toward making the transition to the CPDM. After much consideration of appropriate methodology, the workgroup selected a qualitative approach to the research. They used focus groups, composed of staff who had experienced the transition to CPDM and had been placed at different stages on the developmental continuum, to obtain data. Participation in the focus groups was serendipitously discovered to have a therapeutic effect on the nurses who volunteered to be the subjects for the research study. More description of the staff nurses' experiences is found in Chapter 7.

SUMMARIZING THE TRANSITION

The staff leadership played a critical role in the success of this organizational change. The need for staff leadership development that will advance leadership knowledge beyond the clinical realm and enhance the ability to influence others toward a common purpose was recognized. Under the guidance of the CNE an educational program that teaches the staff nurses the skills necessary to act as a leader was developed. Skills that are taught include negotiation, facilitation, problem solving in a systems framework, and empowerment. As a result, staff has grown in their ability to positively affect both organizational and patient outcomes. The shared leadership program is offered several times throughout the year and is required for those elected to shared governance positions. Additionally, each manager encourages "informal" staff leaders on their unit to attend.

The implementation of CPDM gave us a framework on which to create unity among nursing through a common language that describes practice. This language of CPDM has helped foster a shared nursing experience across the organization.

As for our personal experience in staff leadership roles, we have come to value and respect the ability to build consensus and the wisdom of teams. We have learned that one of the core tasks of leadership is managing uncertainty and coping with fast-changing, shifting environments. We grew to appreciate the strength and resiliency of teams, along with the power and effectiveness of team learning. Our effectiveness as leaders grew as we developed our ability to more fully understand the change process and facilitate decision making in a very fluid and dynamic state.

In addition, we experienced positive changes in our own identities, roles, relationships, and patterns of behavior by virtue of participation in the transition from career ladder to clinical practice development model. We believe this growth is not unique to our personal experiences, but is reflected in others throughout the organization as well.

We have also come to value the rewards experienced through examining our own and others' perspectives and building a shared vision. We now have a peer review system of reward and recognition of nursing practice where the practitioners engage in dialogue and share a common understanding of the contribution of nursing across specialties and areas of practice. Patients move from area to area more smoothly under the collective care coordination of the nursing units, working more as a whole. This has led to an increase in pride and the development of respect for our nursing practice, as well as the desire to nurture and improve practice as new information becomes available. These ongoing efforts mean providing the sort of patient care that supports successful outcomes and acknowledges the work we hold in common.

SUGGESTED READING

Benner, P. (1982). From novice to expert: The Dreyfus model of skill acquisition. *American Journal of Nursing, 82*(3), 403–406.

Benner, P. (1984). *From novice to expert.* Chapter 2. Menlo Park, CA: Addison-Wesley.

DeGroot, H., et al. (1998). Implementing the differentiated pay structure model: Process and outcomes. *Journal of Nursing Administration, 28*(5), 28–38.

Goodloe, L.R., et al. (1996). Clinical ladder to professional advancement program: An evolutionary process. *JONA, 26*(6), 58–64.

Jenkins, J.E. (1996). Moving beyond a project's implementation phase. *Nursing Management, 27*(1), 48B, 48D.

Johnston, B. (1998). Managing change in health care redesign: A model to assist staff in promoting healthy change. *Nursing Economics, 16*(1), 12–17.

Nuccio, S.A., et al. (1996). The clinical practice development model: The transition process. *Journal of Nursing Administration, 26*(12), 29–37.

Porter-O'Grady, T. (1996). The seven basic rules for successful redesign. *Journal of Nursing Administration, 26*(1), 46–53.

Schultz, A.W. (1993). Evaluation of a clinical advancement program. *Journal of Nursing Administration, 23*(2), 13–19.

Staring, S., & Taylor, C. (1997). A guide to managing work force transitions. *Nursing Management, 28*(12), 31–32.

Tonges, M.C. (1997). The whitewater of change: A survivor's guide. *Nursing Management, 28*(11), 64–72.

Wilson, C.K. (1992). *Building new nursing organizations visions and realities.* Chapter 2. Gaithersburg, MD: Aspen Publishers.

Chapter 5

Determining Staff Nurses' Developmental Stages Using a Peer Review Process

Jeanne Smrz DuPont and Barbara Haag-Heitman

Every addition to true knowledge is an addition to human power.

—Horace Mann

As work on the development of the Clinical Practice Development Model (CPDM) neared completion, the methods for its use in promotion and recognition were being formulated. This process was structured and monitored by the Nursing Quality Assessment Council (NQAC). They made an early key decision to use a staff nurse–led peer review process for promotion. Although often espoused as an important professional practice component, the literature lacks examples of authentic peer review as developed at St. Luke's Medical Center (SLMC). The peer review panel became central to the process of promotion using the CPDM. Recognition of each of the staff nurse's developmental stages along the novice to expert continuum through the utilization of a peer review panel came to be known as the "paneling" process. Benefits for the staff participants in the peer review process are widespread. The following testimonial illustrates the enhancement of an individual's professional development as well as on patient outcomes related to participation in the peer review.

My involvement with the novice to expert framework and CPDM began when it was first rolled out at St. Luke's. I wrote my first set of narratives and was staged at the Competent level. My involvement and appreciation of it only grew from there. I have subsequently written two more sets of narratives and have been staged at the Expert level.

I eventually became a panel member to stage others who are going through the process of CPDM. I have participated in that role for two years. Being a panel member has enhanced my practice in various ways. I feel I am a less frustrated and more understanding preceptor since paneling, as I can now clearly understand where new grads "live" in their practice and what can and cannot be expected of them. I believe with that understanding comes the ability to better guide them toward growth and development.

Being a panel member also gives me a sense of connectedness with peers in other areas of the hospital. I feel I better appreciate their practice, and through that appreciation comes the knowledge of available resources and how to access them appropriately.

Reading narratives has also promoted growth in my own practice. I am constantly learning things that I am able to apply to my everyday practice. For instance, I sat on a panel in which a nurse described a patient that developed a retroperitoneal bleed. Having never witnessed one myself, I was fascinated and absorbed the information. A week later one of my patients developed what the doctors felt was a muscle spasm in his lower back. Since the patient had no history of back problems and the pain was acute in onset and severe, I thought back to that narrative and suspected a retroperitoneal bleed. After many attempts to convince the doctors to check for a bleed, they finally agreed to it and the patient did indeed have a bleed. A good catch on my part, but one I wouldn't have made if I hadn't read that narrative one week earlier. I hope to continue my involvement with the novice to expert framework and the process surrounding it that is continually evolving here at St. Luke's, not only to help others, but also to continue to evolve in my own practice.

Courtesy of Ann Wade, RN
Staff Nurse, Med/Surg/Renal

A HISTORICAL LOOK AT PEER REVIEW

The American Nurses Association (ANA) has depicted self-regulation through peer review as an authentic hallmark of a mature profession. Utilization of a peer review process has been evident in the nursing profession for many years with the first American Nurses Association "Guidelines for Peer Review" drafted in 1973. The term *peer* implies a colleague of the same rank and with the same abilities or qualifications (Felton and Swanson, 1995). Nursing peer review has been defined as the process by which registered nurses, actively engaged in the practice of nursing, appraise the quality of nursing care in a given situation in accordance with established standards of nursing practice (Kovach et al., 1985) To assure quality and credibility, performance criteria used by peers in evaluation must be clearly defined and reliably measured (Porter-O'Grady, 1984). Evident in effective peer review is the sharing of power equally and with fluidity among its members. Leadership belongs to the entire peer review group and is shared by the various members throughout the process.

Although often perceived as intimidating and threatening, the value of peer review and focused dialogue around clinical practice offers the many benefits listed in Exhibit 5–1. Opportunities for quality improvement interventions and professional staff development can be identified through peer-focused conversations about practice issues, using the narrative methodology such as CPDM. These conversations create opportunities for nurses to find rich support in their resourceful peer group, a support that has often gone untapped. Determinations of both individual and organizational factors enhancing or impeding service excellence can be attained through examination of peer practices.

Our examination of other promotional models revealed that generally the manager played the gatekeeping role in the decision regarding a nurse's promotional/advancement status. Since our managers' accountabilities were not clinically focused, this approach was not part of the SLMC process. Reflecting on this decision, one of our managers stated, "The fact that clinical peers validate the individual's stage of practice, rather than a nurse manager, who is often more removed from the bedside, emphasizes the value of clinical practice in our organization." The CPDM focused on excellence in practice. Our goal is to stimulate and foster outstanding performance at

Exhibit 5-1 Benefits of Peer Review

- Fosters individual growth
- Affirms and validates an individual's practice
- Recognizes other practice resources within the organization and community that have potential benefits for patients and families
- Identifies alternative styles and strategies for managing problems
- Shares information and strategies for practice
- Helps each other succeed and progress in practice
- Provides a forum for constructive feedback for areas of performance that need enhancement
- Creates opportunities for envisioning professional practice changes to advance the practice
- Provides a sounding board and problem-solving arena for peers
- Enhances a shared understanding of the organization's collective practice, thereby linking the nursing practice community as a whole
- Provides for discussion and development of strategies around organizational and system issues

each level of skill acquisition. Emphasis and value are placed on being the best you can within a developmental stage, rather than on the stage itself. Determination to assure that all the usual Standards of Practice, up-to-date training, and good citizenship criteria are met continues to be handled in the managerial model of annual review. The nurse must have satisfied all the requirements of this annual review before going up for clinical promotion.

These concepts guided the thinking of the NQAC, who structured the composition of the peer review panel at SLMC to include staff nurses whose practice was described by the CPDM framework and who themselves had participated in the panel process as a determination of their stage. Professional commitment, knowledge and skill to assess and give constructive feedback related to nursing practice, combined with good interpersonal and group skills, were essential qualities for those staff nurses engaged in the peer review process.

STRUCTURING THE PROCESS AT ST. LUKE'S

An Implementation Workgroup was commissioned by the NQAC to give structure and guidance for this new process. Using narratives alone as the basis for promotion, with no additional accompanying portfolio-type documentation, was an early and key decision made by this council. Sole use of the narrative methodology clearly focused the intent and purpose of the peer review panel's work. The professional peer appraisal, based on narrative account of the best of practice, is supported by Benner's research on the shifts in perceptions, clinical reasoning, caring practices, and interventions accompanying experiential learning.

Criteria and the method of advancement in the CPDM consisted of the writing of three first-person narrative accounts of current clinical practice by staff nurses with submission to the CPDM peer review panel. These narratives were to reflect patient care situations from within the previous year. The CPDM panel would then meet together and review the narratives. Using a consensual process, they would determine the nurse's stage and forward their recommendation to the NQAC. Applicants during the initial stage of transition had the option of attending an interview with the panel. Feedback from applicants and panel members very early in the implementation process clearly indicated that these conversations around the narratives greatly enriched the process, and the interview quickly became a necessary part of the process. A quality and equitable process was maintained through continuous quality monitoring.

The NQAC reviewed all aspects of the process steps to assure they were done according to the policy set forth. Specifically, they assured that three narratives were submitted and that each panel member was qualified for his or her role. Once assured the quality process was achieved, the NQAC confirmed the panel's stage recommendation and communicated this by letter to both the applicant and manager. Likewise, any deviations from the process were investigated by the NQAC.

Fully understanding the new model and its application to practice was a learning process for the staff and leadership. As would be expected, early in the transition process, the panel observed a somewhat limited understanding of the CPDM by some of their peers. It was not uncommon for early applicants who had not fully explored CPDM to assume that if they had achieved the top level of the old Career Ladder they would naturally be at the top, or experts, in this model. Panel members found that much of the interview time was spent helping the applicant understand the new framework and promotional criteria used for peer review versus celebrating the practice and learning from each other. It was as a result of this learning that the coaching process, as described in Chapter 6, was implemented.

FIRST PANEL MEMBERS

The Narrative Workgroup members were identified as the logical group to become the first CPDM Peer Review Panel by virtue of their in-depth knowledge from the CPDM development, as described in Chapter 3. They were the first registered nurses to be transitioned into the new model in July of 1993.

To participate as a panel member, each Narrative Workgroup member needed to have his or her developmental stage determined using the CPDM framework according to the defined process. Accordingly, each staff RN from the Narrative Workgroup developed three narratives from personal clinical practice. These narratives were reviewed by a panel of three other Narrative Workgroup peers and a recommendation for staging made to NQAC based on the process that had been designed. This review and determination came to be called "staging." Thus the Narrative Workgroup members became qualified as panel members and able to stage other house-wide RN applicants who were applying for placement on the novice to expert continuum.

A house-wide invitation to become CPDM panel members went out to all RNs. Ongoing recruitment of new panel members was also done informally by the peer review panel members through discussion with nurses who expressed interest at the time of their interview at the unit level.

To support new members, the panel composition always included at least one Narrative Workgroup member acting as a resource and mentor. Additional skill and understanding could also be obtained through participation as a silent fourth member of a panel (with permission of the applicant).

Each staff nurse interested in participating on house-wide or unit-based panels was required to go through the staging process individually before being eligible to participate on panels. In addition, all panel volunteers, whether staff nurse, CNS, or manager, had to participate in the validation process. The interest and support was extraordinary and over 150 nurses completed the validation process during this time.

VALIDATION PROCESS

Staff and leadership had been learning about the model throughout its development, and validation packets were developed to determine application of this knowledge.

All panel members need to demonstrate their understanding of the CPDM framework and ability to determine the developmental stage from narratives for all five stages. This validation process includes correctly identifying the CPDM stage, and corresponding domains and individual characteristics of practice within the narrative text. A complete description of the stages and domains are found in Chapter 3.

Validation packets consisted of narratives that had first been collected to assist with the model development. Each potential panel member independently completed a validation packet by correctly identifying the stage and defining characteristics of practice for each narrative. Once completed, these validation packets were scored for accuracy by members of the Narrative Workgroup.

This process of correlating a narrative to a particular stage is demonstrated using the following three narratives.

Narrative #1

I was just beginning the P.M. shift at approximately 1600. There were four other RNs working this shift.

I had an 87-year-old elderly woman, who among other problems was hypokalemic. Her potassium levels had been running low for the last two days since her admission. She had a primary care doctor but was on the Resident Teaching Service, which involved a senior resident and cross-coverage intern. The orders for this patient's meds were written by the resident.

This was the second day that this patient was under my care. Soon after I heard report, I paged through the medication sheets. I knew this patient was on a sliding scale for potassium supplements and had been supplemented with 40 mEq of K+ at 1200 that afternoon. On the second page of scheduled meds, there was a new order written for 20 mEq of K+ that had already been checked off by the previous shift.

This new order for K+ for 20 mEq bothered me since I knew the patient was on sliding scale supplement. I decided to look through the physician's order sheets. There was a sliding scale order for K+ that was written two days previously by the senior resident. Then I looked to see if the new order was written possibly by a different doctor. The new order was written by the intern of the same team. I considered the fact that maybe the intern was not aware of the previous order. I decided to question the intern's new order and make him aware of the sliding scale.

When I paged him, he called back and I stated the situation briefly and asked him if he still wanted me to give the extra dose of K+. He only said, "D/C it."

I felt I had made a good decision in calling the intern. I had to satisfy the nagging feeling that something was wrong, and that I needed to look further.

The most demanding part of the situation was that I was pressed for time and I knew this would use up part of this precious commodity.

I know this is not an example of a life-threatening situation, but I feel that this intervention is part of what nursing is about.

I only hope that if a life-threatening situation would occur, I would have enough experience to recognize it and the time needed to reason it through.

Using the following CPDM definition as a guide, one can determine the focus of this narrative to be consistent with an Advanced Beginner nurse.

Definition: Stage 2 advanced beginners are guided by policies, procedures, and standards. They are building a knowledge base through practice and are most comfortable in a task environment. They describe a clinical situation from the viewpoint of what they need to do, rather than relating the context of the situation or how the patient responds. Advanced beginners practice from a theoretical knowledge base while they recognize and provide for routine patient needs.

In each of the following three examples, the process of coding a narrative using the framework domains and characteristics is demonstrated. The relationship of characteristics of practice from the domains with the text is illustrated. The italicized domains and characteristics follow the bold text that they describe.

I was just beginning the P.M. shift at approximately 1600. There were four other RNs working this shift.

I had an 87-year-old elderly woman, who among other problems was hypokalemic. Her potassium levels had been running low for the last two days since her admission. She had a primary care doctor but was on the Resident Teaching Service, which involved a senior resident and cross-coverage intern. The orders for this patient's meds were written by the Resident.

This was the second day that this patient was under my care. Soon after I heard report, I paged through the medications sheets. I knew this patient was on a sliding scale for potassium supplements and had been supplemented with 40 mEq of K+ at 1200 that afternoon. On the second page of scheduled meds, there was a new order written for 20 mEq of K+ that had already been checked off by the previous shift.

This new order for K+ for 20 mEq bothered me since I knew the patient was on sliding scale supplement. *(Clinical Knowledge and Decision-Making Domain: 1. These nurses are beginning to correlate theoretical knowledge with clinical information. 2. They recognize the importance of knowing about and managing clinical problems. 3. They are beginning to perceive recurrent, meaningful aspects of clinical situations.)* I decided to look through the physician's order sheets. There was a sliding scale order for K+ that was written two days previously by the senior resident. Then I looked to see if the new order was written possibly by a different doctor. The new order was written by the intern of the same team. *I considered the fact that maybe the intern was not aware of the previous order. I decided to question the intern's new order and make him aware of the sliding scale (Collaboration Domain: 3. These nurses are beginning to identify their contributions as members of the health care team.)*

When I paged him, he called back and I stated the situation briefly and asked him if he still wanted me to give the extra dose of K+. He only said, "D/C it."

I felt I had made a good decision in calling the intern. *I had to satisfy the nagging feeling that something was wrong, and that I needed to look further (Clinical Knowledge and Decision-Making Domain: 2. The nurses recognize the importance of knowing about and managing clinical problems.)*

The most demanding part of the situation was that I was pressed for time and I knew this would use up part of this precious commodity.

I know this is not an example of a life-threatening situation, but I feel that this intervention is part of what nursing is about.

I only hope that if a life-threatening situation would occur, I would have enough experience to recognize it and the time needed to reason it through.

Narrative #2: Illustrating the Clinical Practice Development Model Stage 3

Definition: Stage 3 competent nurses integrate theoretical knowledge with clinical experience in the care of patients and families. Care is delivered utilizing a deliberate, systematic approach, and practice is guided by increasing awareness of patterns of patient responses in recurrent situations. These nurses demonstrate mastery of most technical skills, and begin to view clinical situations from a patient and family focus.

Today I was caring for Mr. H, who was progressing normally post–open-heart surgery. He was between seven and nine days post surgery. **I had taken care of him for the past three days on day shift. We had developed a good rapport with each other by the beginning of day four.** *(Caring Domain: 2. These nurses are learn-*

ing to establish and practice within the boundaries of therapeutic relationships.) This day shift started like the others, going into my patient rooms to see how they were doing.

Mr. H was already up and showered. At first glance nothing seemed to be abnormal. I completed a physical assessment and began talking to Mr. H about how he felt and what discharge teaching we could work on that day. Mr. H wanted to tell me something but he wasn't sure how to describe what he was feeling. After several minutes I found he was having an intermittent chest clicking sound, especially at night. When other people were around it never seemed to happen.

At first I thought about Mr. H's history of surgery one year prior and the conversation we had the first day I cared for him. He had told me that his surgeon said the sternum had never healed completely from the first surgery. He had told the surgeon's PA who had assessed him that morning, but had not gotten any satisfaction from his answer. Secondly, *I assured Mr. H that I indeed did believe what he had told me and was going to inform the surgical team of what was happening. (Clinical Knowledge and Decision Making Domain: 2. Providing care based on conscious, deliberate planning.)* I did relisten to heart tones, as I had not heard anything prior. I still didn't hear anything. About 30 minutes had gone by and Mr. H called me into his room because he was experiencing the clicking again. *When I listened this time I heard a very faint clicking.* When I left the room *I found the PA who had seen this patient. I informed him of my findings, but was informed my assessment must be wrong. At first I thought he must be right, as I had never dealt with an unstable sternum before. I checked with the charge nurse and questioned* her about these findings. *I received positive feedback* from her; she felt the sounds I described could indeed be an unstable sternum. *(Collaboration Domain: 1. Recognizing their role and function as members of the health care team.)*

I decided to wait for the surgeon to do rounds and I would make sure he knew about what was going on even if I was going to make a fool of myself. *(Clinical Knowledge and Decision Making Domain: 2. Providing care based on conscious, deliberate planning.)* Several hours had passed and this patient's click was louder and more consistently present now. I also noted that the incision line was not separating but was "bubbling" in a few spots. *I reapproached the PA,* who was again on the floor at this time. *I received the same "You're stupid" look* and was brushed off with the comment that the surgeon would be doing rounds shortly. *(Collaboration Domain: 1. Recognizing their role and function as members of the health care team.)*

Within 30 minutes the surgeon was on the floor. *I followed the doctors into Mr. H's room and listened to them talk about releasing Mr. H the next day.* Mr. H was not going to say anything, *so I needed to speak up. I felt I was putting any credibility I had or would ever have on the line.* (Clinical Knowledge and Decision Making Domain: 5. Assuming an increasing responsibility to advocate for patients and families.) I realized being a patient advocate was more important than what someone thought of me. *I also knew I had to start trusting my nursing judgement and instincts.* (Collaboration Domain: 1. Recognizing their role and function as members of the health care team.) I told the surgeon what I had heard and what Mr. H had told me. He looked at the sternum and listened also. He heard the sternum click and told the PA they were going to have to open the puffed areas and see how unstable it really was. *I stayed with the patient during this and offered as much support as I could.* (Clinical Knowledge and Decision Making Domain: 5. Assuming an increasing responsibility to advocate for patients and families.)

Mr. H's stay progressed to about one and one-half months. Mr. H went to the OR and had surgery to tighten wires and derived a sternal infection that had set in. After this situation I feel I have more confidence in my physical assessments and I realize how important it is for nursing to stand up and become a patient advocate.

Narrative #3: Illustrating the Clinical Practice Development Model Stage 4

Definition: Stage 4 nurses are proficient practitioners who have in-depth knowledge of nursing practice, perceive situations as a whole, and comprehend the significant elements based on previous experience. These nurses demonstrate the ability to recognize situational changes that require unplanned or unanticipated interventions. They respond to most situations with confidence, speed, and flexibility. Progression is from a task orientation to a holistic view of patient care. The nurses develop effective relationships with other caregivers and provide leadership within the health care team to formulate integrated approaches to care. They interpret the patient and family experiences from a perspective that begins to envision and create possibilities.

It is 0830 on a Tuesday morning and one-year-old CW is scheduled for surgery at 0945. The name is familiar, but I cannot place this little girl as I look down the hallway waiting her arrival. I asked the Health Unit coordinator to check with admitting to see if the patient was there. The elevator opens and I recognize the mother with CW in a stroller; CW had undergone a previous procedure a month ago. CW had multiple problems since birth and was undergoing a series of procedures as a result of congenital hand deformation. Mrs. W begins to apologize for being late as she begins to tell me, "CW was choking in the car and I had to pull over to clear her."

As I listened, *I observed no respiratory* distress and asked further questions. *"Has this ever happened before?"* Her response was, *"No, I think she's teething and just had extra saliva* and she was crying so hard she started to choke. I really just had to get her to stop crying but I know she was crying because she was thirsty and hungry from not being fed because of the surgery." *(Clinical Knowledge and Decision Making Domain: 2. Identifies situational changes that require action other than the planned or anticipated.)*

I asked them to follow me to her assigned bed and we began to undress her while I notified surgery of her arrival. The surgery staff had already inquired on the intercom if she was ready to go to surgery as they could take her sooner than scheduled. I turned to the room and asked the mother if she was okay and comfortable with CW going to surgery in light of what had happened today. She had no problem with this and said, "She's really fine, I was just scared driving on the highway trying to get here on time and then having to stop." I reassured her, she was here in plenty of time and we would get her ready at this time.

I began by listening to CW's lungs, which is not routine in the Same Day Surgery Department, but considering what the mother told me, I wanted more of an assessment to inform the anesthesiologist pre-op. (Clinical Knowledge and Decision-Making Domain 1: Perceive the important aspects of a clinical situation and quickly focus in on the accurate region of the problem.) CW was very cooperative and seemed comfortable with the hospital routine. Lungs sounded clear, no respiratory distress, chest movement regular and symmetrical, AP and respirations counted.

I told the mother I would be phoning the anesthesiologist and informing him of the "choking" incidence for her own safety. She seemed comfortable and relieved by this. *The mother requested sedation pre-op for CW as she was sedated previously for surgery and "things went well."* *(Caring Domain: 7. Utilize increasing levels of family involvement and participation in goal-setting, planning, and providing care.)*

I phoned OR room #10 and spoke directly to the anesthesiologist. I told him that the patient had arrived and *I relayed the incident and assessment to him. I also included mother's request for sedation. He was very receptive to this request* and stated, "I did her anesthesia last time and am familiar with the patient." *(Collaboration Domain: 3. Mobilize other health care team members to achieve best possible patient outcomes.)*

I mixed the ordered Versed with apple juice and sweetener. I *gave it to the mother in a medicine cup to give to the child. Mother requested it be put in a syringe as it "works better."* *(Caring Domain: 7. Utilize increasing levels of family involvement and participation in goal-setting, planning, and providing care.)* Mother was then successful to have CW swallow pre-op medication in its entirety.

Mother also requested a sheepskin padding to be placed under the cast as her arm would be secured to abdomen post-op and would avoid rubbing the skin, as it had in the past. *(Caring Domain: 7. Utilize increasing levels of family involvement and participation in goal-setting, planning, and providing care.)* *I wrote a note regarding this and taped it to the front of the chart for the surgeon and OR staff to see. Fortunately, Scott, OR RN, arrived to review the patient's chart and was able to discuss with the mother her concerns. (Collaboration Domain: 2. Develop effective relationships with other caregivers and provide leadership within the health care team.)* Scott went to patient's room and reassured the mother and assured her he would discuss appropriate padding with the surgeon for post-op.

The anesthesiologist arrived as CW's eyelids became heavy and the mother was rocking her. After a brief conversation, he carried CW to surgery.

CW's mother related she knew this would be a long surgery (estimated time four hours) and she was going for something to eat before going to the waiting area.

I was approached in my department by a representative from the Home Care Agency, who requested I give respiratory supplies to

Mrs. W. I needed to question her more regarding why such supplies were needed. She explained that CW had needed respiratory care at home since birth. This information had not been recorded on the database or in the History and Physical. I informed the representative that the mother was in the waiting area, if she would like to take them to her. Her response was, "That would be great, I have never met her." So I took her to the family waiting area and made the appropriate introductions. Both women seemed glad to meet each other and were still visiting 20 minutes later as I passed the area discharging another patient.

CW returned after a short stay in PAR and was then given apple juice per her mother's request. I noted a sheepskin pad in the crib and assessed a small square had been cut from it and was placed under CW's casted arm with supporting sling to adduct her arm. I told her mother she could take home the excess sheepskin to use as needed. She was very appreciative of this.

CW met our discharge criteria, other than being a little sleepy, within a half hour. ***Mrs. W verbalized her anxiety about being discharged as early as possible as she didn't want to drive a lot in the city rush hour traffic.*** I phoned a progress report to the anesthesiologist for approval for discharge per mother's request and he agreed as long as the mother was comfortable with the child. ***I favored discharge ASAP,*** knowing Mrs. W was experienced with taking care of CW after numerous surgeries. *(Caring Domain: 5. These nurses recognize that healing requires more than physical interventions. They promote an environment grounded in empathy, kindness, and deep regard for the individual. Patient and family strengths are identified and possibilities are recognized.)*

I had a feeling of satisfaction as Mrs. W pushed CW in the stroller to the exit for discharge. I met CW's needs as a surgical patient but was also able to relate to Mrs. W and saw a change from anxiety to relaxation in our ambulatory department. I thanked Scott (OR RN) as I saw him later in the day for the reassurance he had given the mother pre-op and following through with the suggested padding to the surgical site.

Candidates needing additional skill development working with the narratives participated in narrative workshops facilitated by the Narrative Workgroup. A second validation packet was completed and scored in the same manner. One-on-one sessions were held for anyone needing further skill development until validation could be completed.

CREATION OF HOUSE-WIDE AND UNIT-BASED PANELS

All staff nurses were required to make the transition from the Career Ladder into CPDM within a seven-month time period. Chapter 4 discusses the organization's commitment to this time frame. To facilitate completion of the staging process for over 700 Registered Nurses, the Implementation Workgroup recommended establishment of both house-wide panels and unit-based panels.

House-wide panels were responsible for all RN applicants applying for Proficient and Expert, stages 4 and 5. Unit-based panels were responsible for RN applicants applying for Advanced Beginner and Competent, stages 2 and 3. Exhibit 5–2 outlines the qualifications and expectations of the CPDM panel members.

To reduce anxiety and feelings of vulnerability during the transition process, it was an option to request that one panel member be from the applicant's specialty area of practice (i.e., ambulatory, cardiac). As we gained experience with the model, both panel members and applicants found that specialty representation was not necessary for understanding the practice described in the narratives. As nursing as a whole grew in its trust and understanding of comparable nursing practices and concerns across practice areas, the specialty representation option was discontinued. For developmental purposes, the sharing of narratives within the specialty is encouraged so that others may benefit from the clinical wisdom evident in them. Exhibit 5–3 illustrates how the panel composition has evolved since transition.

PANEL FACILITATOR ROLE

There is a trained facilitator for every peer review panel who acts as the chair of the panel. Coordination of the panel process

Exhibit 5-2 St. Luke's Medical Center, Milwaukee, Wisconsin, CPDM Housewide Panel Pool Member Qualifications and Expectations

---

I. Housewide Panel Member Qualifications.
   A staff RN who has:
   A. Been confirmed by the NQAC as a Stage 4 or Stage 5
   B. Supported the philosophy and process of CPDM
   C. Been validated in identifying the Characteristics of Practice within narratives.

II. Housewide Panel Member's Role Expectations

   A. Availability and skill maintenance
      1. Will participate at least twice a month until transition into the CPDM process is completed.
      2. Exhibit flexibility to sign up for either morning or afternoon times to meet panel needs. *Sign up for specific dates/times through the PNA secretary.
      3. Will panel or complete a self learning validation packet at least once every three months in order to maintain their skills.
      4. Is not eligible to participate in formal coaching.
      5. The panel will be selected from available panel members. You may call the PNA office to verify if you are on a panel.

   B. Come prepared to the panel review by:
      1. Identifying the Characteristics of Practice in the margin of your copies, and
      2. Identifying any potential interview questions you might have.
      3. Avoid looking at the stage applied for until you have reviewed the narratives and made your own recommendation.

   C. If you as a member have any concerns with the process or the written narratives, contact NQAC chairperson in advance of the panel review as soon as possible.

continues

Exhibit 5-2 continued

> D. Participate in the panel review process:
>   1. Come on time and keep on schedule.
>   2. Maintain confidentiality.
>   3. Promote an atmosphere of respect, teamwork, and growth.
>   4. Promote a positive experience for the applicant.
>   5. Support the role of the facilitator.
>   6. Work toward consensus.
>   7. Keep discussion related to CPDM framework.
>
> E. Assist the facilitator in filling out the FACILITATOR SUMMARY FORM and other required documents after each applicant's panel process is completed. The facilitator will ask for the following information:
>   1. Summation of major consensus points.
>   2. New Characteristics of Practice that were identified.
>   3. Any barriers to delivering nursing care that were identified.
>
> F. Confidentiality
>   1. Confidentiality is inherent to all aspects of the process.
>   2. Hand in all narratives and notes to the facilitator for shredding.
>   3. If approached by the applicant for further feedback in a situation where the panel was not in consensus, or where the panel and the applicant did not agree, refer the applicant to the facilitator.
>
> Signature: _____Date: _____
>
> *Source:* Courtesy of St. Luke's Medical Center, Milwaukee, Wisconsin.

(e.g., record and time keeping and communication with the NQAC) is the essential component of the facilitator role. Another important role of the facilitator is to maintain the flow of the dialog during the panel review by encouraging participa-

Exhibit 5-3 Evolution of Panel Composition

Initial Implementation	Post Transition

3 Members
  Minimum of 1 staff RN
  at Expert Stage
  Other members may be at
  Proficient or Expert Stage
  1 CNS or Nurse Manager
  (acts as facilitator)
	3 Members—All Staff
	  Minimum of 2 staff RNs
	  at Expert Stage
	→ Other member may be at
	  Proficient or Expert Stage
	  1 staff member is trained
	  facilitator

Specialty Representation—
  optional
	→ Specialty Representation for
	  appeals only

House-wide panels for
  Proficient and Expert
  Promotion
Unit-Based Panels for
  Advanced Beginner and
  Competent Stages
	→ All House-wide Panels

tion of all panel members, while they work toward group consensus around the staging decision. The facilitator is also responsible for clarifying communication and keeping an open dialogue during and after the panel interview. The facilitator is an experienced panel member who has completed our Facilitator Training workshop, which is designed for participants to attain additional skills related to giving feedback, achieving group consensus, negotiating conflict, and performing other duties related to the role. Mentoring new panel members is another responsibility of the facilitator. Facilitator qualifications and role expectation are further described in Exhibit 5–4.

While panel members were learning these new skills during the transition process, the CNS and Nurse Managers performed the facilitator role, as the necessary skills were inherent in their existing roles already.

Exhibit 5–4 St. Luke's Medical Center, Milwaukee, Wisconsin, CPDM Housewide Panel Facilitator Qualifications and Role Expectations

Facilitators will meet all qualifications and role expectations of the CPDM panel members.

I. Qualifications

A staff nurse who:
A. attended facilitator training
B. demonstrates ability to communicate clearly and negotiate conflict
C. demonstrates ability to reach group consensus
D. demonstrates the ability to accurately articulate and document characteristics of practice within all of the domains in the panel review
E. is experienced as a panel member.

II. Role Expectations

A. Ensures the integrity of the panel process by:
   1. keeping discussion related to the CPDM Framework
   2. facilitating panel members to remain focused on characteristics of practice
   3. providing timely feedback to panel members as needed, e.g., regarding appropriateness of comments and questions
   4. ensuring uninterrupted time of panel review

B. Communicates any concerns regarding the integrity of the panel process to NQAC via Facilitator Summary Form and notification of NQAC or designee:
   1. in advance of panel review
   2. within 24 hours following panel review and interview

C. Documentation
   1. coordinates transcription of specific characteristics and respective stage of practice in the margins of the original copies of the narratives

continues

Exhibit 5–4 continued

> 2. includes succinct reference words as appropriate
> 3. documents interview questions on narratives
> 4. completes all forms
> 5. collects working copies of the narratives from the panel members and has them shredded
> 6. forwards forms and narratives to PNA office at least 24 hrs before next NQAC meeting
>
> D. Appeal Panel
>   1. the facilitator will disclose to the panel members prior to interview that this is an appeal.
>   2. emphasizes confidentiality and that no prior communication between the two panels has occurred
>   3. ensures that all appeal and nonconsensus panels reach consensus, since a 3rd panel review is not an option
>
> *Source:* Courtesy of St. Luke's Medical Center, Milwaukee, Wisconsin.

COORDINATION OF THE PANELING PROCESS

All applications and supporting narratives are submitted to a central location for scheduling and processing. The application form and process steps are shown in Exhibits 5–5 and 5–6. Panel members and facilitators indicate their availability in a centralized CPDM scheduling book. Generally within two weeks following receipt of the staff nurse's application and narratives, a panel date is scheduled. The PNA secretary coordinates the process of duplication and distribution of the applicant's narratives to each panel member along with the location and time of the scheduled panel. Typically, one panel is scheduled to stage two to three applicants per session.

To assure that communication about the panel is timely, notification about the interview date, time, panel location, and facilitator's name is done through the U.S. mail.

Exhibit 5–5 CPDM Application Process

A. Write three narratives (see narrative criteria on front of application).
   1. Employee # and Narrative # should appear on each page of each narrative.
   2. Number the pages of each narrative (Page 1 of 4, Page 2 of 4 etc . . .).

B. Utilize a validated coach to discuss characteristics of practice present in narratives and strategies for continued growth.

C. Complete application form, including coach and manager signature.

D. Retain a personal copy.

E. Completed packet should be mailed in an interdepartmental envelope to the PNA office by the 15th of each month.

F. Await notification of panel date and interview time.

G. Attend interview

H. Receive verbal feedback from facilitator of panel regarding recommendations.

I. Receive final notification of stage from Housewide Nursing Quality Assessment Council.

Source: Courtesy of St. Luke's Medical Center, Milwaukee, Wisconsin.

PANEL NARRATIVE PACKET

Each panel member receives the applicant's packet of three narratives along with the application indicating the applied-for stage prior to the panel date. Panel members independently read the narratives and identify the CPDM stage and characteristics of practice that are present for each of the three. CPDM characteristics are identified in the margins next to the defining text.

To prevent any potential biases while reading the narratives, the applicant's name is blinded to all but the panel facilitator. Narratives are identified by employee ID number only.

Exhibit 5-6 Application for CPDM Staging/Advancement

Name: _____ Unit:_____Shift:_____

Address: _____ City:_____
Type of Application: Initial: _____ Start Date: _____
Advancement: _____ Appeal: _____

Date of Last CPDM Confirmation: _____

Narrative Criteria:
   Narratives submitted must meet the following criteria:
   a. typed standard size and print
   b. double spaced on 8 1/2 × 11 inch paper, one side only, and one inch margins
   c. length may vary but a maximum of 5 pages per narrative is preferred
   d. number each page of each narrative 1, 2, 3 in upper right hand corner of each narrative
   e. name on application form only
   f. employee ID number on each page of all three narratives. No applicant name on or within the narratives

PANEL SPECIFICS:
Would permit a silent 4th panel member: Yes_____ No_____

PANEL TIME:
All applicants will participate in a 30 minute interview. Preferred time: 0800-1200 □   1200-1600 □

I understand that my narratives may be utilized by any of the governing PNA Councils when systems, process or quality issues are identified. In addition, I give permission for publication of my narratives: Yes_____ No _____ (This may or may not include my name)

---

continues

Exhibit 5–6 continued

Manager's Signature_____
Date_____

Applicant's Signature_____
Date_____

Coach's Signature_____
Date_____

FOR PNA OFFICE USE: Date received_____ Initials_____
      Application Complete: Yes_____ No_____
      Comments: _____

Source: Courtesy of St. Luke's Medical Center, Milwaukee, Wisconsin.

Although available, most panel members also disregard the applicant's applied-for stage until they have made their own determination.

On the scheduled panel date, the members gather and each applicant's set of three narratives is reviewed by the panel together for a maximum of 45 minutes. Group discussion centers around the CPDM domains and characteristics found in the narratives. Identification of interview questions that would enhance the panel's understanding of the nurse's stage is done. A possible stage recommendation is also discussed and compared to the applicant's self-staging.

Once the initial narrative review process is complete and just prior to the applicant's arrival for interview, the facilitator reveals the applicant's identity to the panel members. The applicant is then invited in for the interview. Initially the conversation around practice was not a required part of the staging process. It was quickly recognized that without this forum, affirmation and validation of an individual's practice was not possible and neither was there a sharing of clinical wisdom and practice strategies. The interview quickly became a necessary component. This decision is discussed in detail in Chapter 9.

APPLICANT'S INTERVIEW

The true essence of peer review begins with the dialogue around practice at the interview where the benefits of peer review can be realized. Each interview is approximately 30 minutes in length. The applicant is welcomed by the facilitator and introductions are made of all panel members. The panel's work reviewing the narrative is explained to the applicant, as well as what to expect during the interview. The applicant is informed that the panel has formulated some interview questions to guide the discussion, but the discussion is not limited to these questions and they should share any other aspects about the narrative situations they feel appropriate.

Typically, each panel member facilities the discussion around one narrative. This technique encourages the participation and ownership of the process by each member. When the interview is completed, each applicant is asked to step out of the room for a brief period of time to allow the panel to incorporate the new information from the interview into their final recommendation. This recommendation of the stage incorporates information gained from the panel narrative review as well as the interview and is a panel consensus decision. The recommendation for staging is based on the presence of the CPDM characteristics from all three of the CPDM domains of caring, clinical knowledge and decision making, and collaboration. When the applicant rejoins the group, the facilitator communicates the stage recommendation to the applicant. The power of the peer-to-peer dialogue, with subsequent learning, is illustrated in the following reflections from a panel facilitator.

> The entire process, going through it as an applicant, being part of the panel pool, as well as now being a facilitator for the panel process, has been invaluable for me in my clinical practice and professional development. I have been able to grow in my knowledge of the entire process and see firsthand how nurses in a variety of set-

tings have grown their practices as well. I have learned a great deal and plan on continuing to learn, not only about others' practices, but about myself.

Initially I had gotten involved with this entire process after I had been staged during transition. I had been skeptical at first and wanted to find out more about the entire process.

My staging had gone well. I had been both excited and nervous. My coach felt the same. I wondered how three nurses that I had never met would be able to evaluate my practice based on my three narratives. When the panel welcomed me and I sat down, I didn't feel threatened at all. We discussed my narratives. I wasn't grilled for clinical knowledge. I felt that they really did see my practice through the questions they asked and the way that the discussion was led.

After I was staged, I was even more curious as to how this process worked and took the initiative to become part of the panel pool. As I began reading narratives, the characteristics of practice became much more evident. Although not perfect, the model appeared to fit the development of nurses regardless of what area of the medical center they worked. Now as I read through the narratives, I can automatically pull out characteristics.

As part of the panel pool I feel that I have grown immensely in my practice through others sharing their narratives. The experience is unbelievable! I have encouraged every applicant that would qualify to also become a part of the panel pool. The first few times that I had sat on the panels, I was nervous. Was I finding the same characteristics that the other members would find? I soon found how amazing the process was! Although each of us had the narratives on our own and pulled out the characteristics individually, we came together and found identical characteristics in identical places. It was as if we were all reading from the same comments.

This doesn't always happen. There have been times when all three panel members don't see the same characteristics or even the same stage. This is why the dialogue is so important. We are responsible for coming up with appropriate discussion areas and open-ended questions for clarification to allow the applicant to expand on the situation and enlighten the panel. This is done without leading the applicants or making them feel like they are being grilled.

Many applicants facing their first panel have commented on how they were fearful and somewhat intimidated and envisioned that they were going to be sitting at the far end of a long table with the panel members at the other end asking intimidating questions. They seem to visibly relax once they have been introduced to the panel members and the process is explained to them.

It is always challenging when an applicant decides to apply for a stage much higher than his or her narrative supports. The panel works extremely hard to come up with open-ended questions to help pull out characteristics that the applicant may have alluded to in the narrative without having the applicant feeling he or she is being examined under the microscope. I have been on panels wherein, after much discussion, the applicant has been staged lower than the applied-for stage. I have been prepared for the questions and comments that often follow this situation, only to hear the applicant say something like, "I knew that I was a stage lower, but I thought I would go for broke."

It seems to me that most applicants really do understand the process and they value it.

I have taken to noticing the behaviors of others outside of nursing and I find myself automatically thinking about their developmental stages. I can see this framework being used in a large variety of situations and professions and feel it is a good way to help individuals continuously grow within their areas along the developmental continuum.

Courtesy of Janet L. Rewolinski, RN
Staff Nurse, Surgery Center

APPLICANT AND PANEL MEMBERS' RESPONSES

Individual responses can range from joy to dissatisfaction. Chapter 7 details the research done on the staff experience. When clarification of the recommendation is needed, the CPDM framework is used as the basis for discussion. The facilitator supports the applicant while upholding the panel's recommendation. Not all panel decisions are consistent with the applied-for stage, as some are higher and some are lower. Applicants not satisfied with the recommendation are offered information about the following options: the appeal process, application for promotion in six months, and/or referral back to the coach. The appeal process is rare and used less than 1 percent of the time. Details of our experiences with panel outcomes are described in Chapter 9.

At closure of the interview, the facilitator provides a written reference sheet for the applicant, as shown in Exhibit 5–7. Included is the panel stage recommendation and an NQAC contact person. Following the NQAC staging confirmation, the applicant receives a copy of his or her narratives with the consensus CPDM characteristics and interview questions documented in the margins. This validation process is concrete and respectful of the practice presented. It is the sharing and celebration of practice with peers that helps connect individual nurses to the whole body of nursing, as illustrated by an operating room nurse's reflection on the peer review process.

> In surgery it is easy to become isolated behind closed doors to the various nursing practices. I feel I gain an incredible amount of knowledge and valuable insights by reading the narratives of other nurses. I am occasionally asked by my peers, "How do you know that?" The answer is through knowledge gained through my paneling experiences.
>
> Some surgery nurses have told me that they feel that they may not be able to demonstrate the Caring domain of CPDM, since their exposure to the awake patient is of short duration. I have found in paneling that just the opposite is true. Surgery nurses stage high in the Caring and Collaboration domains. If anything, they may be more challenged to demonstrate their Clinical Knowledge and Decision Making.
>
> Although I am a surgery nurse, it is easy for me to identify characteristics of practice in all types of nursing. When I panel I identify the same characteristics of practice as the other panel members.
>
> I have found that narratives are a valuable part of the promotion and advancement process.
>
> Courtesy of Jennifer Cooper, CNOR
> Staff Nurse, Surgery

SUPPORTING PANEL MEMBERS

During transition phase, panel member group debriefing sessions were held on a regular basis. These informal sessions created a forum for problem-solving and for learning about and sharing strategies to support the applicant and panel process,

Exhibit 5–7 CPDM Panel Applicant Information

30 minutes of interview time is allotted. This can be recorded as meeting/inservice time charged to your own unit.

We are recommending to Nursing Performance Improvement Council (NPIC) that your narratives demonstrate the characteristics of practice found in Stage _____.

NPIC will consider this recommendation at their next meeting on _____.

You will receive written notification verifying NPIC confirmation of your stage within two weeks of the above date. Please contact the PNA Secretary if you have not received notification.

Your feedback is very important to us, and will assist us in our ongoing review of the CPDM process and facilitate policy changes and educational opportunities as needed.
Take a few minutes now, to complete the Applicant Feedback Form, enclose it in the envelope provided and place in the NPIC envelope on the interview door.

Please contact the NPIC chair, if you have any concerns about your CPDM panel process.

Comments:_____
_____
_____
_____
Facilitator:_____ Date:_____

Source: Courtesy of St. Luke's Medical Center, Milwaukee, Wisconsin.

particularly around giving feedback. A deeper appreciation of the clinical wisdom embedded in the narratives was also realized through the sharing done at these meetings. These conversations substantially enhanced the development of all panel members' skills and knowledge about the CPDM and nursing practice at St. Luke's. Confidentiality of all individual applicant and panels information was maintained.

There was much learning during this transition time. Adaptations to the entire process occurred under the direction of the NQAC, which was also undergoing a transition from a quality assessment to a performance improvement council. Maintaining the integrity and quality for the CPDM promotion process fell within this council's domain and is detailed in Chapter 9.

REFERENCES

American Nurses Association. (1983). *Peer Review in Nursing Practice.* Kansas City: Author.

Felton, G., and Swanson, E.A. (1995). Peer review. *Journal of Professional Nursing*, 11, 16–23.

Kovach, J.S., et al. (1985). *Peer consultation in a group context: A guide for professional nurses.* New York: Springer.

Porter-O'Grady, T. (1984). *Shared governance for nursing, a creative approach to professional accountability.* Rockville, MD: Aspen.

Chapter 6

Coaching: An Integral Component

Alice Kramer

In helping others succeed we insure our own success.
—William Feather

LEARNING RELATIONSHIPS

Three methods are commonly used to assist staff nurses in their professional development: education (formal and informal), experience, and learning relationships. These learning relationships include precepting, mentoring, and coaching. Learning relationships are the bridge between education and appropriate application experiences in the work setting. According to Yuki (1989), relationship skill "seldom receives the attention it deserves from leaders preoccupied with immediate problems and crises" (p. 286). Most leadership and career development occurs informally and produces variable and unpredictable results. Despite its potential for staff and organizational enhancement, relationship skill development remains a neglected process in many organizations.

Although both large and small corporations acknowledge the importance of mentoring, coaching, sponsoring, and role modeling for the development of their next generation of leaders, it seems doubtful that many are doing a good job in this regard. In light of the changing health care environment, leaders need to pay particular attention to learning relationships and to clearly understand their differences. Precepting, coaching, and mentoring are separate and distinct activities that influence staff and the organization in different ways.

Learning relationships for career development can be viewed as occurring on a continuum in which precepting is at the low end, mentoring at the highest end, and coaching exists somewhere in the middle. Precepting is a relationship in which a nurse assists the less experienced nurse by explaining the context of the work environment, articulating the norms of professional practice in that particular area, making introductions among the peer group, and being available to answer work-related questions. This relationship is usually a short, formal, institutionally mandated pairing of individuals. It is instrumental in nature, meaning that tasks are focused on role expectations and behavior (Everson, Panoc, Pratt, and King, 1981; Limon, Spencer, and Water, 1981; Shogan, Prior, and Kolski, 1985).

Mentoring is on the higher end of a learning relationship continuum because it incorporates more intense time and emotional commitment than precepting or coaching. Mentoring occurs when a senior person with experience and position provides information, advice, and emotional support for a junior person, in a relationship lasting usually over several years. The hallmarks of mentoring are the duration of the relationship and the power differential of the parties involved (Yoder, 1990).

Coaching is an ongoing, face-to-face process of influencing behavior by which the coach (peer or supervisor) and the employee collaborate to achieve increased job knowledge, improved skills in carrying out job responsibilities, a stronger and more positive working relationship, and opportunities for personal as well as professional growth. By its nature, this relationship has a greater psychosocial component than precepting, but it is still less psychosocially intense than mentoring (Concilio, 1986; Shore and Bloom, 1986; Stowell, 1988; Thomas and Kram, 1988).

The concept of coaching evolved out of a sporting context. The coach is concerned with helping each athlete reach full potential and encouraging the athletes to work as a winning team. Gallway (1975), a Harvard educator, posited the proposition that the "opponent within one's own head is more formidable than the one on the other side of the net" when referring to the "inner" obstacles of coaching the tennis player. If a coach can enable a player to reduce or eliminate these internal obstacles to performance, then an unexpected natural ability would flow forth without the need of much technical help from the coach.

Applying this to a managerial perspective, Whitmore (1995) states, "Coaching is unlocking a person's potential to maximize their own performance—a process of bringing out the best in people. Ability will emerge providing the performer can be freed from the inner doubts, uncertainties and fears that they harbor in the relation to their own performance."

LEADERSHIP'S ROLE

Maximizing staff's potential and performance via coaching is quite timely given the changes in health care and the expectations that nurses be leaders. As Naisbutt and Aburdene (1984) state: "The dominant principle of organization has shifted from management (once needed in order to control an enterprise) to leadership (now needed to bring out the best in people and to respond quickly to change)...to lead one must learn to coach, inspire and gain other people's commitment. The new workforce of the 1990s will help your company achieve its objectives if it can achieve its own personal objectives as part of the bargain."

A recent study by Yoder (1995) suggested that if nurses perceived that an interest was being taken in their professional and career development and that they felt valued by a developer, then usually the relationship was viewed as professionally important. This perception of importance often influenced nurses' clinical development and their intent to stay in a positive environment. The study concluded that coaching was perceived by qualified nurses as the predominant mode of valuing in terms of professional development.

ENHANCING PROFESSIONAL GROWTH THROUGH FOCUSED PRACTICE DIALOGUE

St. Luke's Medical Center (SLMC) has a strong commitment to the professional development of staff nurses at the point of service. It has had a fully integrated shared governance system since 1992 wherein nurses define and are accountable for their own practice. SLMC began a process of Shared Leadership development in which administration, management, clinical nurse specialists, and staff nurses are developing their understanding and ability to share the accountability of decision making with the point-of-service providers.

It is sometimes assumed that nurses desire to "move up" within an organization by leaving direct service nursing for management or administrative positions. Based on the findings of Yoder's study (1995), nurses were very concerned about working in an environment that values quality nursing care. They were not necessarily interested in moving out of direct clinical practice toward management positions. Similarly, nurses at SLMC wanted to create a system that valued their contribution with patients, families, and their colleagues in collaborative practice at the bedside.

In 1990, St. Luke's Medical Center had just gone through a process wherein staff nurses were seeking a more effective means of defining and developing their clinical practice, as well as a means for measuring and recognizing that practice. Much of nursing's finest contributions were not visible to the organization, and individual nurses were not being recognized for their caring, clinical knowledge and decision making, or collaborative skills. Advancement was based on a traditional career ladder, which was limited predominantly to citizenship and nonclinical activities. As a result of these limitations, nurses created the Clinical Practice Development Model (CPDM), grounded in Patricia Benner's novice to expert model. Inherent in the CPDM process is the ability of staff nurses to engage in dialogue regarding their clinical practice. This necessitates an environment in which nurses feel comfortable and safe in sharing their thoughts and feelings about the intimate nature of their practice. It also requires an organizational climate of shared responsibility for the demands, resources, and constraints of good practice encountered in the organization. This means that when breaks in good practice occur, they cannot be assumed to be the sole responsibility of any one practitioner. Revelations about individual practice are assumed to have, in addition to the individual contributions, collective and structural contributions. Since the practice of nursing is shared by many nurses in a particular organization and culture, individual stories describe that shared practice as well as individual practice. Narratives uncover strengths and vulnerabilities of the nurse and the organization. The interpretive focus must be on ways to extend and reward excellent practice. Strategies to strengthen and develop the practice through education and attention to organizational structures and processes that could impede practice must all be attended to. Narratives revealing vulnerabilities of individuals must *not* be seized upon as sources of blame and punishment. Making the relational aspects of nursing practice visible opens up the possibility of improving the organizational supports for the central relational areas of nursing practice. But this visibility must not be misunderstood as opening up the organizational possibility of mandating, or standardizing, nurse-patient relationships. Minimal standards of courtesy, effectiveness, and respect can be required, but supportive advocacy requires more than can be demanded or even promised outside the particular nurse–patient/family relationships.

In 1993, St. Luke's Medical Center developed a system of formal coaching for clinical development and recognition that added value to the preceptorship, informal/unstructured coaching, and mentorship that already existed within the organization. Administration at SLMC set the tone for valuing learning relationships with its intense investment in the resource use of clinical nurse specialists (CNS) and nurse managers in the coaching process. Coaching required extensive time and skills that were already consistent with their role functions and skill levels. At the time of implementation, SLMC had in place over 20 CNSs and 15 Nurse Managers who demonstrated strong communication/feedback skills and were experienced in observational skills and performance evaluation. Their role accountabilities at that time gave them credibility to offer clinical insights, provide constructive criticism, and facilitate learning with the staff nurses. The CNSs demonstrated expert clinical practice and consultative skills in a wide array of patient populations.

Each clinical unit at SLMC, both inpatient and outpatient, has access to a CNS and a Nurse Manager. Together they have created a collaborative dyad approach to staff development and performance improvement. While the Nurse Manager has fiscal and resource responsibilities, the CNS has clinical responsibilities for professional development. Whereas the manager is generally more involved with counseling activities that are issue- or problem-focused, the CNS is more engaged in practice discussions that are clinical and educational in nature.

LEARNING THE COACHING ROLE

Although SLMC had developed a large resource pool of coaches with strong clinical and communication skills, CPDM challenged this group to develop additional coaching skills within the context of the novice to expert continuum. Since narratives were the main vehicles for dialogue about clinical practice, specific skills of identifying behaviors and characteristics of practice within the narratives needed to be learned. These are not simply intuitive skills. They need to be developed.

In July of 1993, SLMC began the implementation of the CPDM for over 700 nurses. At that point, prepared by some formal education sessions, CNSs and Nurse Managers began to coach staff nurses. Coaches partnered with staff nurses who were on the panels that formally reviewed the narratives and recommended the stage designation to the Nursing Performance Improvement Council. True to Peter Senge's principles of a learning organization (1990), SLMC designed a variety of team learning experiences and shared vision exercises for the panel members, coaches, and shared governance leaders to participate in together. Initially they all attended the same didactic sessions, which included interactive opportunities to discuss narratives, and observed simulated paneling. A videotape was developed to enhance consistency with interpreting characteristics and communicating them within a coaching or paneling session. Coaches and panel members were required to complete validation packets (see Chapter 5), which measured the accuracy with which they could identify characteristics of practice in the narratives and correlate them to various stages of the CPDM framework. One of the most valuable learning experiences for coaches was to participate or observe the actual paneling experience. This reinforced the congruence between coaching and the panel experiences.

Although coaching was not a required component of the process initially, word of mouth quickly spread that there were distinct advantages to having a dialogue about one's narratives and staging before one went to the actual panel review.

Staff nurses have always had the option of choosing their own coach, sometimes even using more than one. Still today, the majority of staff tend to use the CNS on their unit as their coach because of the CNS's awareness of their clinical practice; often there is a prior learning relationship. Some staff preferred the objectivity and perhaps a different perspective of less familiar coaches by utilizing CNSs from other units.

During the nine-month transition to the CPDM model, a small number of CNSs and managers were also members of the paneling process. This made those people ineligible to function as both the coach and a panel member for the same staff nurse because of the obvious conflict of interest. Once transition was completed, the paneling process became entirely a function of staff nurses, and the CNSs and select managers who chose to remain in that role did coaching. In the beginning, coaches were literally learning as they went, relying on their inherent skills and the mentoring of other experienced coaches. Initially, the core group of leaders of the CPDM project underestimated the learning curve required of both staff and coaches in understanding the model. This included writing narratives and correlating skill acquisition and characteristics of practice along a novice to expert continuum. Staff and coaches alike needed actual experience in writing and reading clinical narratives. Unfortunately, the accelerated nine-month pace at which the process was being implemented allowed some staff to write only the same three narratives that they would use for staging. They would have benefited by more opportunities to read and write narratives for the sole purpose of learning the process and exploring their practice. Instead their experience was limited to narratives that had significant implications for status and salary range related to placement on a clinical development continuum. The qualifications and expectations of coaches were formally integrated into policy and procedure in 1994 after transition (see Exhibit 6–1). As coaches gained in knowledge and experience, they pooled their insights into a list of suggested coaching guidelines.

Exhibit 6-1 Coaching for CPDM Staging/Advancement Qualifications and Expectations

---

    I. QUALIFICATIONS
        A. CNS/NC
        B. Nurse manager
        C. Select Stage 5 staff nurse as negotiated with nurse manager and CNS/NC.
        D. Select Stage 5 staff nurse not presently serving as a member of the housewide panel pool.
        E. Validated in their ability to read clinical narratives and identify characteristics of nursing practice based on CPDM framework.
        F. Demonstrates strong communication skill with giving constructive feedback and managing conflict.

   II. EDUCATION
        A. Objectives
           The coach will be able to:
           1. Define basic coaching ground rules (guiding principles)
           2. Identify logistics, flow and dynamics of the coaching process, which prepares applicant for staging/advancement

---

continues

Exhibit 6–1 continued

3. Identify characteristics of clinical practice within narratives based on the CPDM framework
4. Demonstrate coaching skills of giving constructive feedback and managing confusion and resistance
5. Describe outcomes of successful coaching
6. Differentiate their coaching role from the other role accountabilities of CNS/NC, nurse manager or staff nurse
7. Suggest strategies to promote growth along the continuum of novice to expert

B. Method
1. Individual sessions with CNS/NC using a variety of educational strategies
   a. didactic written information and dialogue
   b. role playing
   c. videotapes
   d. joint coaching session(s) with staff nurse who plans to apply for staging/advancement
   e. observation of the paneling/interview/staging process

III. ACCOUNTABILITIES
A. Accountabilities of New Coach
1. New coach (Stage 5 staff nurse)
   a. contact manager and CNS/NC to negotiate coaching role with consideration of:
      1) actual number of staff that will pursue initial staging or advancement in the next year
      2) existing coaching resources already available to your unit
   b. plan developmental strategies with CNS/NC
   c. work with CNS/NC to accomplish objectives as stated
   d. charge coaching time to your unit as (02X)
2. New coach (CNS/NC, manager)
   a. contact CNS/NC to plan developmental strategies
   b. work with CNS/NC to accomplish objectives as stated

continues

Exhibit 6–1 continued

    B. Accountabilities of CNS/NC Mentor for New coach
       1. Works with new coach to assist in meeting the objectives as stated
       2. Notifies NPIC chairperson in writing that the RN has met all the criteria to function as a coach for the CPDM process
    C. Maintaining Coaching Skills
       1. When approached by an applicant to be his/her coach, consider the length of time since your last coaching experience
       2. If it's been >3 months since reviewing narratives, complete a self-learning validation packet obtained through PNA office
       3. Seek out formal/informal opportunities with your colleagues to enhance your coaching skills as needed
IV . SUCCESSFUL COACHING
    A. Criteria for Successful Coaching
       1. Positive change in performance and/or renewed commitment
       2. Achievement or maintenance of a positive work relationship
       3. Mutual, communicates respect, problem-focused, change oriented
       4. Follows an identifiable sequence or flow with specific communication skills
    B. The Outcomes of Successful Coaching are:
       1. Positive change in performance
       2. Achievement or maintenance of a positive work relationship
       3. Mutual discovery
       4. Respect
    C. A Coaching Process:
       1. Is satisfying to the employee
         -Logically (objective, meaningful)
         -Psychologically (have sense of closure)
       2. Is interactive

continues

Exhibit 6–1　continued

> 3. Proceeds through interdependent stages
> 4. Employs specific skills
>
> *Source*: Courtesy of St. Luke's Medical Center, Milwaukee, Wisconsin.

COACHING GUIDELINES

Following are anecdotal comments from experienced coaches.

- Consistently use language of the CPDM framework to give it real and practical meaning.
- Give feedback that is descriptive, not judgmental or punitive; specific, not general.
- Focus on nurse's behavior, not basic character traits.
- Focus on internal validation and self-reflection rather than on external validation of the stage or "grade."
- Express concern for helping the nurse develop his or her full potential, while valuing practice at each stage of development (avoid comparison to other staff nurses).
- Be open, gentle, and patient. These narratives are an intimate portrayal of a nurse's professional life.
- Be aware of each applicant's learning style and be flexible in strategies to educate and facilitate.
- Self-assess own communication style (step back and see self in action; observe effects).
- Help applicant develop own sense of self and own practice, and recognize need for development. Help applicant find satisfaction in the efforts to explore and grow into practice.
- Emphasize each one's personal accountability to engage in this process and find own meaning for self.
- Utilize open-ended, reflective questions to stimulate the writer's thinking.
  - What were you thinking at the time . . . feeling at the time . . .
  - Can you talk/write more about that...
  - Why did you do that...decide that...

- - Tell me why you chose to write about this particular situation . . .
  - What you're *telling* me is not as clear in your *written* description...
  - What was your role/contribution to this situation...as a nurse...
- Be careful not to contaminate/color their stories with your own perspective/bias.
- Don't tell the applicant to change his or her story. The narrative is uniquely his or her own and is reflective of individual practice. If you have someone who is excited about what he or she has done but you are clear it is not expert performance, acknowledge what the applicant did do and ask if this narrative is representative of day-to-day performance. You wouldn't want to add your own ideas or interventions to embellish another's story.
- Advise the applicant to write in the first person, past tense (other styles of narrative writing have an awkward feel and can become confusing). Assist with grammar and spelling but don't change the words. Words chosen to describe situations offer valuable insights into performance and development.
- Translate local language (i.e., NSVD means normal spontaneous vaginal delivery) to ensure that panel members will easily understand the story.
- Avoid any information that could identify the patient, family, or staff involved.
- Don't guarantee them that your coaching will get them the desired stage designation that they are seeking. Rather, guarantee them that your coaching will help them express themselves more fully about the situations.

Although a specific coaching class was developed, the greatest wisdom generated was most often from informal dialogue between the coaches and with panel members.

Another prevailing concern for coaches during transition/initial implementation was time constraint. Coaches needed to invest significant amounts of time in developing their skills of interpreting narratives. The amount of time and energy expenditure in actual coaching sessions was also substantial. CNSs did approximately 90 percent of the initial coaching during transition and each CNS coached at least 20 staff; some coached over 50 staff nurses. However, this provided a wealth of experience with narratives, and as a group, their skill level, confidence, and effectiveness increased exponentially.

Initially, many narratives were succinct, more like case studies filled with isolated pieces of data. Dialogue with a coach assisted the nurse in better understanding the complexities of each clinical situation, helping to embed it in written narrative. Interpersonal, ethical, and clinical judgment, with collaborative aspects of actual practice, were explored and better captured in the written narratives. Well-developed narratives provided a means to see the quality and depth of nursing practice.

An example of coaching might be: A nurse initially wrote, "The family was ready to see their father now that he had died. I tried to make it okay for them. They stayed about 20 minutes and left." After the coach asked questions about what the staff nurse's understanding was of this family's grief experience and what her specific nursing interventions were, the nurse wrote, "The wife was looking stoic but the daughter was sobbing and clinging to her mother. I moved the patient to a quieter area in the unit so the family would not feel rushed or on display. I turned the lights lower and made sure that Mr. B was as presentable as possible. His face was clean of blood and emesis. I made sure that his hands were exposed and the side rail was down so that the family could touch him if they wanted."

Another nurse described her activities following the stillbirth of an infant. "I took footprints, pictures, and a lock of hair to give to the family." After the coach inquired about the importance of these interventions and their relation to the patient's entire experience, the nurse revealed her deep knowledge and understanding of the perinatal grief experience. She went on to describe, "Creating memories for the family of their baby is an important part of making the experience real and meaningful. The family usually leaves the hospital without the benefit of having their friends and family having seen the baby, so the

loss seems invisible. Families have told me about the importance of these memories to them after they leave the hospital."

The coaching process during 1993–1994 was often more
time-consuming than present day because everyone was learning this new system and staff nurses came to the coaching session with limited readiness to identify their own characteristics
of practice in advance. Today, nurses that are seeking advancement are educated to the model, to their responsibility, and
to the role of the coach prior to their first coaching session.
They are coming prepared with much higher levels of understanding of the CPDM framework and with narratives quite
fully developed.

Throughout the transition period of initial staging, coaches
identified concerns regarding some staff's lack of understanding
and accountability to learn about CPDM. Some staff truly valued the new direction and approach of the novice to expert
model, while most were unsure but willing to engage in the
struggle to understand it. There were also those staff who were
extremely resistant to "buying in" to this model. A major role
for coaches, both during transition and ongoing, is to educate
staff and attempt to reframe negativism into opportunity for
professional clinical growth. Coaches have to quickly demonstrate concrete evidence of the ability to see characteristics of
practice within written narratives that correlate directly to the
CPDM framework. This helps the process become real to the
staff nurse and begins to give everyone a common language of
characteristics and specific behaviors to discuss practice.

ESSENTIAL ELEMENTS

Over the year, coaches and staff have frequently attempted to
define successful coaching. Some criteria usually mentioned are
the fostering of authentic dialogue, free exchange of information and ideas, and a climate of collegiality, respect, and trust. It
is essential that both the coach and staff nurse are mutually
involved in the process. The language of the CPDM framework
used by the coach also needs to be clear and understood by the
staff nurse. Appropriate feedback by the coach hopefully gener-

ates energy in staff nurses who are motivated to improve and grow their practice. They gain more clarity about the performance expectations as they relate to the novice to expert continuum. Staff nurses have expressed more satisfaction in their efforts to change as they increased their understanding and ability to visualize characteristics of nursing practice that have developed.

Both the coach and staff nurse need to have the same understanding and expectations of their roles during the coaching session(s). The coach conveys a concern to help the staff nurse develop to full potential and the staff nurse assumes personal accountability to write accurately about practice, understand the framework, and engage in a dialogue to assist in revealing their practice in the narrative. The coach's role is to explore the staff nurse's clinical practice and assist in the most accurate revelation of that practice within the narratives. Coaches are challenged to demonstrate exquisite listening and conflict resolution skills when there is significant discrepancy between the assessments of development by the coach and the staff nurse.

Ideally, successful coaching results in the staff nurse and coach being relatively congruent in their perceptions of the applicant's practice as revealed in the dialogue and written narratives. The staff nurse can make an informed and insightful declaration of a stage based on self-assessment and the coach's feedback. The applicant then feels prepared for the panel/interview process and has a clear understanding of the framework as the basis for the panel's stage recommendation. Despite any discomfort or conflict within the coaching session, both the coach and staff nurse should have achieved and should now be able to maintain a positive work relationship. Ideally, the staff nurse has received affirmations of his or her practice and will continue to utilize the coach for ongoing professional development.

Coaches celebrate with the staff nurses when they have been staged at the level that is acceptable to the staff nurse. Personal forms of congratulations and public forms of validation within the unit or across the organization are utilized, depending on what is comfortable to that individual staff nurse. Coaches console staff nurses whose paneling outcome has been disappointing, and they assist them with the interpretation of panel feedback. In both cases, the coach continues in learning relationships and developmental plans with the staff nurses for life-long learning.

SLMC has utilized a formal evaluation mechanism throughout the CPDM process. The feedback from coaches and applicants related to coaching have focused on certain themes. Currently applicants report high levels of knowledge about the framework and preparedness for the panel. Coaches report a strong degree of consistency between their identification of the characteristics of practice with the applicant and panel's recommendation of staging.

In the years since implementation of CPDM, the process of coaching has continued to evolve. CNSs continue to do the majority of the coaching. In select situations where coaching resources were limited, select nurses at the expert stage have also been encouraged to assume the coaching role. However, given the large resource pool of CNS, only a few staff nurses are currently functioning in the coaching role. The majority of staff nurses that are interested in a formal role with CPDM are functioning as panel members and facilitators on the house-wide panel. CNSs had a wealth of experience with narratives during initial transition to CPDM. Since that time, some coaches have had significantly fewer opportunities to coach, especially if the staff on their unit is predominantly staged at 4 or 5 and there are few outside hires to their unit that require initial staging.

In 1996, some of the coaches were able to do high-volume coaching again because of a merger of SLMC with another hospital. Over the course of nine months, approximately 150 RNs were coached and staged. Unlike our initial experience, CNSs who had no prior relationship with the staff did the majority of coaching. Every attempt was made to give the staff options regarding their coaches and to direct them to the CNSs who had familiarity with their practice specialties.

FOSTERING PROFESSIONAL DEVELOPMENT AND LIFELONG LEARNING

Some observations made by the coaches were as follows:

My experience is that with each coaching session, I felt that I became rejuvenated (re-energized) with CPDM. I guess that I have never experienced this before. It was as though each opportunity provided more excitement for me to share with upcoming staff for coaching, almost reconfirming for me this is what nursing practice is about and how CPDM is truly played out within my unit.

Mary Schmidt, 1998

What was clear from the beginning is that the integrity of the process would only be maintained if the individual staff nurse took accountability for engaging in the staging experience. As both a coach and panel member at the time it was a kind of 'immersion therapy'—a seemingly endless learning experience about the model, the process, myself, and the nurses I worked with. Communication between coaches, panel members, applicants, and facilitators supported all of us as we grew in our respective CPDM roles. I remain convinced that the model truly represents the novice to expert philosophy as it is lived at SLMC. Other things are different, though. There is a genuine excitement exhibited by nurses who are promoted in the model. Coaching is an expected process with a formal beginning that is not time limited. The role of the CNS in staff development and leadership is, in part, legitimized by the coaching role. All of these things are benefits of the model that I had not anticipated. In summary, CPDM has probably done more to enhance my job satisfaction and strengthen my role as a unit-based CNS than any other process I can recall.

Sandra Menting, 1998

The Clinical Practice Development Model has been a timely strategy to assist nurses at SLMC in their professional development, given the changing expectations within health care and the emphasis being placed upon nurses as leaders (Andrews, 1993; Dean, 1995; Thomas, 1995; Yoder Wise, 1995). This model has been consistent with St. Luke's commitment to valuing learning relationships such as coaching.

SLMC has integrated the principles of Senge's (1990) learning organization and continues to invest in a series of programs designed to enhance the staff nurses' ability to share in the leadership at the unit level. Clinical nurse specialists and managers, as coaches, partner with staff nurses to integrate the concepts of the novice to expert model for professional development and positive patient outcomes.

For lifelong learning to be relevant and valued, it's essential that individuals engage in dialogues involving critical analysis of assumptions/mental models and explorations of alternative meanings (Mott, 1992). Coaching helps the staff nurse to be a reflective practitioner and promotes creative exploration through collaboration and dialogue, thus fostering critical and creative analysis. Coaching assists staff nurses to unlock their potential to maximize their own performance. Helping them to learn, rather than teaching them how, enhances their own professional development.

As characteristics of practice are revealed in the narratives, they can be discussed using the common language of the novice to expert model. The characteristics are used as indicators of a nurse's level of performance. This provides an incredibly useful "road map" for professional development, making the personal action plans of staff nurses far more specific. There has been an emerging clarity of performance expectations for nurses as they develop along the novice to expert continuum. Utilization of CPDM has helped create direction and focus for the development of all nursing staff at SLMC. Coaching has been an integral component of that process.

> The rewards and benefits of coaching are tremendous. The authentic dialogues around practice and commitment to the individual development of the staff are transformational. With each interaction I learn more about both the practice and the individual. The narratives reveal the true nature of the staff's work, which is profound. I have experienced a range of emotional responses including great pride, joy, and sadness, to the situations they share with me in their narratives. This deeper understanding and connectedness to the staff and practice helps guide my work as a CNS at the individual, unit, and organizational level. Indeed, the coaching process can be challenging in terms of time and energy, as the interaction with staff

is sacred and demands that you be fully present with the nurse in this experience. Sessions must be free of interruptions and require putting aside all other organization demands. My conversations with the staff about practice using their narratives has given me valuable knowledge and insight that was not readily available before. Working with the staff in this new way is truly the most important and satisfying work I have ever done.

Courtesy of Barb Haag-Heitman, 1998

REFERENCES

Andrews, M. (1993). Importance of nursing leadership in implementing changes. *British Journal of Nursing, 2*(8), 437–439.

Concilio, R. (1986). Will coaching pay off? *Management Solutions, 31*(9), 18–21.

Dean, D. (1995). Leadership: The hidden dangers. *Nursing Standard, 10*(12–14), 54–55.

Everson, S., Panoc, K., Pratt P., and King, A. (1981). Precepting as an entry method for newly hired staff. *Journal of Continuing Education in Nursing, 12*(5), 22–26.

Gallway, T. (1975). *The inner game of tennis.* London: Jonathan Cape.

Limon, S., Spencer, J., & Water, V. (1981). A clinical preceptorship to prepare reality based ADN graduates. *Nursing and Health Care, 2*, 67–269.

Mott, M. (1992). Developing key players. *Journal of Nursing Administration, 22*(6), 54–58.

Naisbutt, H., & Aburdene, P. (1984). *Megatrends 2000.* London: Futura Publications.

Senge, P. (1990). *The fifth discipline.* New York: Doubleday.

Shogan, P., Prior, M., & Kolski, B. (1985). A preceptor program: nurses helping nurses. *Journal of Continuing Nursing Education, 16*, 139–142.

Shore, L., & Bloom, A. (1986). Developing employees through coaching and career management. *Personnel, 63*(8), 34–41.

Stowell, S. (1988). Coaching: A commitment to leadership. *Training and Development Journal, 42*(6), 34–38.

Thomas, L. (1995). A programme for nursing leadership. *Nursing Standard, 10*, 12–14.

Thomas, D., & Kram, K. (1988). Promoting career enhancing relationships in organizations: The role of the human resource profession. In M. London and E. Mone (Eds.), *Career growth and human resource strategies* (pp.49–66). Westport, CT: Greenwood Press.

Whitmore (1995). *Coaching for performance–a practical guide to growing your own skills*. London: Nicholas Brealey Publishing.

Yoder, L. (1990). Mentoring: A concept analysis. *Nursing Administration Quarterly, 15*(1), 9–19.

Yoder, L. (1995). Staff nurses' career development relationships and self-reports of professionalism, job satisfaction, and intent to stay. *Nursing Research, 44*(5), 290–297.

Yoder Wise, P. (1995). *Leading and managing in nursing*. Baltimore: Mosby Year Book, Inc.

Yuki, G.A. (1989). *Leadership in Organizations* (2nd ed.) Englewood Cliffs, New Jersey: Prentice-Hall.

Chapter 7

Staff Nurses' Experiences During Transition and Beyond

Barbara Haag-Heitman and Susan Nuccio

Discovery consists of looking at the same thing as
everyone else and thinking something different.
　　　　　　　　　　　　　　　—Albert Szent-Gyorgi

As with all transitions, there are those who embrace and
welcome the changes and those who are hesitant or
maybe even resistant. The staff extended their caring
practices to each other during this time and were sensitive to
each other's experiences. Many nurses came forward to lend
their support. The following account illustrates this behavior.
This nurse also encourages seeing beyond the current experience of transition and recognizing greater possibilities.

Letter to Editor of the *Interchange*
All of us may be skeptical at some time. The novice to expert
model seemed to blossom out of nowhere for some of us, and for others, well, we watched it develop with interest and intrigue. For years,
nurse managers and educators were left the responsibility of assuring that the nursing staff provide care at an "expert" level. For some
that meant providing safe and "competent" care, for others it held a
completely different meaning.
　　And this may describe the way most nurses at SLMC feel about
the Clinical Practice Delivery Model (CPDM)...it holds a *different*
meaning for each of us. But I want to share with you my belief that the

137

model does describe individual practice, that it does allow for creativity, individuality, and *specialty* within nursing practice. CPDM speaks a universal language. More important, it is a means of self-assessment and self-awareness.

It is a brave step we are all taking, exposing ourselves to our colleagues. Narratives may be very personal, as nursing should be. No wonder it makes us feel a bit uncomfortable to share. So imagine taking the next step—sharing your narratives with a national organization and complete strangers who would scrutinize them further. That's what I did . . .

When I was staged by my panel in September 1993, I met with three peers, one a unit representative. They agreed with my evaluation of my practice and I was confirmed at the expert stage 5. More importantly, I had the opportunity to discuss my practice with my colleagues. I shared details about the nursing care I had given to others. During the interview I realized that though we may "share stories" with our colleagues each day, we don't always look at the meaning of the story or what we learned from the event. We don't always take that opportunity to assess the care we gave and evaluate its effectiveness. And yet that's what we need to do in order to grow as individuals and as professionals.

So I decided to test the system further. If indeed my colleagues felt my practice to be at an "expert" level, then too should a panel of national representatives, right? RIGHT! I submitted my narratives to the American Association of Critical Care Nurses Awards Program. I applied for the AACN/3M Excellence in Critical Care Clinical Practice Award. Recently I learned that I am a recipient of the award.

So why do I bring this all up to you now? Well, I think the award speaks to the fact that CPDM does work, it is recognized on a national level, and it does reflect one's own practice. The award truly illustrates my professional goal in my practice as a critical care nurse. It also serves to validate my practice, much like a panel of my peers did, not long ago. I am very proud to represent SLMC and the Greater Milwaukee Area Chapter of AACN at the National Teaching Institute in Atlanta this May as a recipient of the award. But I'm not telling you all this to toot my own horn, I wanted this opportunity to congratulate all of you who have taken the step to be transitioned into the CPDM model. And I applaud all of you who are going through the process now. Give the model a chance to help you see your nursing practice in a new light. I assure you it will be an opportunity for both personal and professional growth.

Courtesy of Lori Hislop, RN, BSN, CRN
Staff Nurse, Thoracic Transplant ICU

STUDY PURPOSE AND METHODOLOGY

The Nursing Research Council (NRC) recognized that along with this major shift in our promotional process, new cultural norms and expectations for nursing practice were being established. We were interested in understanding the range and variation of the staffs' experiences during the transition as well as learning about the critical factors that influence nurses' perceptions during significant organizational changes. This information would give us insight that would be useful in shaping the posttransition process as well as in preparing for future organizational changes.

Thus, a workgroup was called to develop a study that would capture staff's perceptions of their experiences. The clinical nurse specialist who was a member of the Research Council was designated as the workgroup leader. She solicited nursing staff volunteers along with several clinical nurse specialists, a patient care manager, and the Director of Nursing Education as workgroup members.

An exploratory, qualitative research design, using the focus group method with content analysis, was used for the study. The focus group method was selected because its efficiencies of time and resources enable it to obtain the viewpoints of many nurses in a short period of time. The focus groups were conducted in April and May of 1994. Staff nurses from Stages 2 (Advanced Beginner) through 5 (Expert) who had completed the CPDM transition process prior to the end of March were invited to share their views and perceptions. A list of nurses who completed the CPDM process was maintained by Human Resources. The list was sorted numerically by unit area number and alphabetically by nurse's name. The researchers, choosing every third eligible nurse from every nursing unit, systematically identified potential participants. The secretary from the Nursing Research Center was trained in focus group screening process by the research team. She called the staff nurses on their clinical units and conducted a screening telephone interview using the Screening Filter detailed in Exhibit 7–1. Four focus group sessions were held, with nine being the average number of nurses attending each session. Each focus group lasted approximately two hours. A trained moderator and assistant

Exhibit 7-1 Screening Filter

RNs Who Have Completed the CPDM Transition Steps at St. Luke's Medical Center

Interviewee Name_____ Date_____

Unit_____ Unit Extension Number_____

Hello, my name is _____, and I'm calling for the Nursing Research Council at St. Luke's. We are conducting a short survey of the nurses who have completed the CPDM transition steps and I would like to ask you a few questions. The questions will take less than 2 minutes. Is it OK to begin?

1. Have you received notification of your confirmed stage from NQAC?
   ( ) Yes   [CONTINUE]
   ( ) No   [TERMINATE]

2. At what stage were you confirmed?

   ( ) Stage 2   [RECRUIT 6]
   ( ) Stage 3

   ( ) Stage 4   [RECRUIT 6]
   ( ) Stage 5

3. Overall, how would you describe your perception of your experience? More as a positive experience or more as a negative experience?
   ( ) More positive   [RECRUIT AT LEAST 6]
   ( ) More negative   [RECRUIT AT LEAST 6]

[PARTICIPANT RECRUITMENT]
_____, the Nursing Research Center at St. Luke's is sponsoring a focus group with nurses who have completed the CPDM transition steps to share their ideas and opinions about

---

continues

Exhibit 7–1 continued

their transition experience. We know that you are busy but we
need to understand the individual nurse's actual CPDM transition experiences. We would like you to join a group of other
clinical practice staff nurses as we discuss this topic. The meeting
will last about an hour and a half. No one else in the group will
be from your clinical area. You will be reimbursed at your hourly
rate for the time that you are in the focus group. This is not an
evaluation of your practice, but strictly a research project to evaluate the CPDM transition process. Are you interested in participating?

( ) Yes   [CONTINUE]
( ) No   [THANK AND TERMINATE]

Four groups will be held from mid April to early May in the
Environmental Services conference Room on the 8th Floor at St.
Luke's. The dates and times that are available are . . .

Source: Courtesy of St. Luke's Medical Center, Milwaukee, Wisconsin.

moderator conducted each session. Each session was audio-
taped. All participating nurses chose a pseudonym, which was
used in conversations during each session.

Informed consent and demographic data were collected prior
to the start of each focus group. The moderator's purpose was to
guide the group through a questioning route outlined in
Exhibit 7–2 and to facilitate participation by all group members. The assistant moderator's purpose was to record notes so
that the speakers could be identified by code with their comments when the audiotape was transcribed. The research team
developed the questions for the focus groups. General questions about the nurses' experiences with the Clinical Practice
Development Model transition process were used at the beginning of the session. This allowed each nurse to talk and adjust
to the group. The questions were designed to become more specific as the session progressed.

Exhibit 7-2 Guide for Focus Group Questions

1. All of you here have completed the CPDM transition steps from a career ladder level to a stage in the clinical practice developmental model. As a way to get started, tell us about how you felt about your nursing practice when you practiced under the career ladder.

2. Now, tell us about your experience in going through CPDM transition.

3. Let's discuss how you feel about the experience. Was it a pleasant or unpleasant experience?
   Probe: What factors were most important in making the experience positive?
   What factors were most important in making the experience negative?
   (If not raised by the group, probe for the importance of each of the following):
   a. Choosing the event of the narrative
   b. Writing the narrative
   c. Coaching
   d. Looking at the framework
   e. Deciding your stage
   f. Interview
   g. Agreement/Disagreement or acceptance with panel's staging
   h. Written follow-up by NQAC
   i. Recognition
   j. Self-reflection
   k. Dialogue with others

4. If you could change the transition experience in any way, what would you change?
   Probe: How would this change make a difference?

5. Some of you state that you had positive experiences while others had negative experiences. Do you see any differences in the process of transition that might have led to these different experiences?

continues

Exhibit 7–2 continued

Probe: Why do you think these differences exist?

6. Now think about your current nursing practice. What effect has your CPDM transition experience had on the way you feel about your nursing practice now?
 Probe: What makes you say this? Can you give us an example of how your practice is different? or the same?

7. What is the most important effect that transitioning to CPDM has had on your nursing practice? (If not raised by the group, probe for the importance of each of the following):
 a. Recognition aspects
 b. Reward
 c. Responsibility
 d. Job satisfaction
 e. Change in practice
 f. Cultural norms
 g. Expectations in nursing practice
 h. Unit cohesiveness

8. Is there anything else about your transition experience that you would like to share that we have not yet touched upon?

Source: Courtesy of St. Luke's Medical Center, Milwaukee, Wisconsin.

The tapes from the focus groups were transcribed. The typed text was given to the research team for analysis. The focus group tapes were summarized and coded using content analysis procedures described by Krueger. Data management was facilitated by technical support from the Ethnograph software program. Members of the research team independently and then as a group coded the transcripts to detect recurring themes. Research team meetings were held to derive a consensual summary of the findings. The team reached consensus of the recurring themes, definitions, and subcategories based on words used by the participants to describe their experiences of transition.

RESULTS OF THE STUDY

A variety of responses to the transition were discovered in the focus group discussions. The learning of one of the participants helps illustrate these findings.

> During our conversion from a career ladder to the novice to expert model, I was able to participate in a focus group. The purpose of the focus group was to talk about the participants' personal experiences with the conversion. I remember being struck by the wide range of experiences and emotion.
>
> The very personal nature of this professional conversion was obvious. For some, writing narratives had been as easy as a chat at break. For others, it was equivalent to sharing an intimate experience with a total stranger. Sharing our professional experiences revealed as much about who we are as what we do.
>
> Concerns related to writing and language abilities were the basis for a great deal of discomfort. Some felt that lack of skill in these areas would not lead to the professional validation deserved. Others felt that strong skills could lead to validation at a professional level not yet evident in daily practice. This was a challenge for the whole process from coaching to panels.
>
> The personal experiences shared with the group related to coaching and panels revealed a lot about our ability to seek and receive feedback about our professional practice. It also revealed that both coaches and panel members were growing in this process. Internalizing the model and developing the skills to guide participants successfully through the process required experience and personal growth.
>
> Participating in the focus group was a great experience for me. I learned that this process was different for each of us. That our experiences in the process are as unique as we are as individuals. I also learned that my professional growth and personal growth have been more closely linked than I ever thought.
>
> Courtesy of Sherry Levenhagen, RN
> Staff Nurse, CVICU

Six themes emerged from the focus group data and describe movement from the singular, personal effects of the experience toward a connection to the whole through supportive relationships. These themes are listed along with excerpts of their supporting comments in Exhibit 7–3. The nurses' perception of how the process influenced nursing practice ranged from a

Exhibit 7–3 Themes and Supporting Comments

Feeling the individual effects of the transition process

"I didn't see before that there are so many ways I could improve my nursing practice, new things I could incorporate."

"One of the most difficult parts was laying my practice out on paper and saying, 'Okay, this is what I do and you are going to judge it.'"

Understanding the transition process

"When I sat on several panels, that's when I got the understanding of what the framework was all about."

"I wasn't sure what I was supposed to be writing about. Once I met with my coach, she gave me guidance with that."

Getting through the transition

"It was helpful to have access to a coach."

"I wrote about things that really had an impact on a patient or a family."

Critiquing the credibility of the transition process

"This is providing a language for nurses to talk about their practice."

"I was impressed how the staging criteria could be drawn out specific to mental health."

"The people who were on my panel had taken a lot of time to actually study my narratives."

Feeling the group effects of the transition process

"I got recognition from my manager and CNS . . . . the pin, the letter, and I think we had lunch too. That was very nice."

"Now that everyone's through it, nobody talks about it."

Participating in the focus group

"This was very enlightening to hear how others felt in the process."

---

somewhat limited focus on its individual effect to a more systemic view, as shown in Figure 7–1.

Strategies to help nurses prepare for continued advancement through the peer review process in the posttransition phase were also identified. One of the recommendations suggests seeking opportunities for self-reflections, introspection, and professional growth through the use of journaling, a mentor relationship with an expert nurse, or by seeking continuing education opportunities. Seeking experiential learning opportunities to expand one's clinical knowledge to evaluate one's personal growth along the novice to expert continuum is another recommendation. An example of how one unit continued their dialogue and growth beyond the transition period is described:

> Since the inception of the CPDM process six years ago, we have often thought of it as an evaluation and a promotional tool, and that is of course how we primarily use it. But our practice is continually growing, even if we *have* been a nurse for 15 or 20 years, and have achieved the expert stage on the continuum. On our unit, we have taken CPDM a step further, challenging ourselves to grow our practice.
>
> I work on a busy women's health unit, consisting of GYN surgicals and oncology (including chemotherapy administration), pediatrics, general female medical, and overflow mom-babies from the nearby OB unit. This number of "specialties" creates a challenging work environment.
>
> About a year and a half ago, a fellow RN and I started what we have termed "Shared Learning Experiences." Every other month or so, a group of stage 4 (proficient) and 5 (expert) nurses meet to discuss patient scenarios. We take turns presenting our patient situations (similar to a narrative, only in verbal rather than written form), and then leading a discussion around the situation. We have met at work as well as at one another's homes. Meeting at each other's houses gives a more informal feeling to our get-togethers; however, meeting at work enables those working on the unit that day to come in and join us, even if only for 15 minutes. Discussions have ranged from the technical aspects, such as managing difficult clinical situations and showing how we networked with other units and disciplines on these issues, to moral-ethical dilemmas. We also have explored

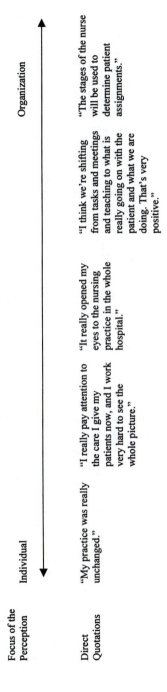

Figure 7-1 Nurses' perceptions of the effects of CPDM transition on their nursing practice

Source: Courtesy of St. Luke's Medical Center, Milwaukee, Wisconsin.

the essence of caring and giving support and facilitating decision making with a young woman dying of cancer, and her family.

Such discussion serves to "uncover" each other's practice. It also forces us to reflect on our *individual* practice, and how we would have reacted in the same situation. It challenges all those participating to raise our high standard of care just a bit higher.

We started our sessions with the proficient and expert staged nurses, but lately have invited all the nurses to join us in some sessions. These sessions help encourage their growth and help them to "see the bigger picture" as they progress in their practice.

Our future goal is to host some interdepartmental sessions, for instance, since we have GYN oncology patients on our unit, we would like to invite nurses from the main oncology unit to present and discuss a case with us.

Courtesy of Judy Hunholz, RN
Women's Health

Although not captured formally in the research study, we were aware that experienced staff were concerned about how their staging would translate to other areas if they transferred. With time we learned to trust a nurse would still remain at the same stage if time was allotted for skill development. One nurse's experience with this is described in her story.

I have been an RN for almost 16 years. For 15 of those years, my main focus was obstetrics and gynecology. About six months ago, the opportunity arose to broaden my horizons to also include a pediatric focus.

I was concerned about how I would do in an area I had such little experience in. My pediatric background was limited to the newborns and teens I cared for in obstetrics and the experience I have had with my own two children. I did have one semester of pediatrics in nursing school, but that was over 18 years ago. Needless to say, my first few months in the Pediatric clinic have been very humbling. I went from being the experienced resource person and preceptor in obstetrics to the orientee in pediatrics. I am always having to ask questions, look things up in textbooks and resource manuals, watch how to do things, etc. I am beginning to feel a bit more confident with my skills and knowledge of pediatrics as the weeks go by, but I know it will be a long time before I reach the point I had achieved in OB.

I was talking to one of my peers a few weeks ago, and we were discussing my feelings related to my new position in the clinic. She pointed out something very interesting to me that is helping me a great deal in my transition. She acknowledged that even though my knowledge base regarding pediatric issues may be limited, the *quality* of care I provided, and the *way* I deliver that care, reflects my expertise and the dedication I have to my patients and to nursing in general, no matter where I am practicing. In my concern over not always knowing the right answer or having to ask to be shown how to carry out a certain task, I underestimated my own abilities. As I look back over situations that have occurred in the clinic over the past few months, I am now able to identify many times where I responded not as an orientee, but as a nurse drawing on 16 years of valuable experience.

> Courtesy of Laurie Kadunc, RN
> Staff Nurse

The value of talking about and defining one's practice by participating in dialogue sessions or focus groups to explore the meaning of the CPDM was also evident. Assisting staff with their practice growth and development requires discovering the strategy that will best suit them as individuals. Positive and supportive relationships can help individuals achieve new insights and grow in new ways. One staff nurse's struggle with the narrative methodology and subsequent growth from his self-reflection is shared in the following story.

When I heard of the new process for validating our practice, I thought my colleagues had lost their minds. Writing a story to demonstrate my level of practice seemed laughable and embarrassing. My concern was that other professionals, such as doctors and lawyers, use more objective information to measure their practice. They rely on mortality and morbidity rates or number of cases won versus lost to demonstrate their level of practice. I felt that narratives were too subjective to yield an accurate measure. I was also concerned that writing ability would be too significant in the process. One of my greatest concerns was that other professionals would not take us seriously if we used stories to measure our expertise.

I was very vocal in my opposition to this new system and was able to rally quite a few supporters. Our plot to block the new system included a plan to wear black armbands to meetings to demonstrate our displeasure and solidarity. We had a journalist unfamiliar with health care draft a narrative to disprove the reliability of the system. We tried everything we could think of to stop the madness.

Eventually our pleas were silenced when the system was approved and set in motion. Desiring to remain employed, I wrote my narratives. I felt that over time the flaws of the system would surely be revealed and we could abandon it at that time.

While writing my narratives, I became aware of gaps in my practice that I hadn't seen before. This was a very effective means of personal evaluation. Although I staged at the top level, I was able to identify areas where my practice could improve. I also realized how effective I was in some very difficult situations. This was reinforced when I shared some of my narratives with colleagues at a conference. The speaker asked for stories from the audience, and since my narratives were fresh in my mind, I shared them. I was overwhelmed by the positive reaction I received.

That's when it hit me. I finally understood how narratives could work. Storytelling is one of the oldest forms of communication. Much of history was passed on in this manner. For storytelling to have lasted this long there must be something to it. I realized two people could tell a story of the same event and have very different stories based on their level of understanding. That is what is evident in a narrative. By the way, the narrative written by the journalist was staged at the level of the nurse who supplied the information.

This self-evaluation, prompted by writing my narratives, led me to enroll in graduate school the next semester. I recently graduated and am now coaching others to write their stories and reveal their practice.

Courtesy of Tim Heyse, RN, MSN
Staff Nurse, CICU

SUMMARY AND RECOMMENDATIONS

These study findings suggest that we have been successful at shifting the focus of recognition to direct patient care, as was the original intent of the CPDM. Additionally, we learned we were able to identify the following organizational strategies, which could be used to positively influence other major organizational changes.

- Provide resources, support, education, and time for change process
- Shift educational paradigm to support novice to expert educational strategies (i.e., appropriate blend of didactic instruction, experiential learning, computer-assisted instruction, mentorship)
- Redesign nursing care delivery model
- Create an environment for professional growth along novice to expert continuum
- Provide resources for focus groups and dialogue sessions
- Be supportive of staff members' expressions of feelings
- Provide education of leadership staff to manage change
- Allow realistic time frames for the transition process to occur
- Facilitate individual achievement of professional goals (i.e., tuition reimbursement, flexible scheduling, expert clinical nurse resources)

Full results of this study have been published in the *Journal of Nursing Administration* (Nuccio, 1996).

REFERENCES

Nuccio, S.A. (1996). The clinical practice developmental model: The transition process. *Journal of Nursing Administration, 26*(12), 29–37.

SUGGESTED READINGS

Krueger, R.A. (1988). *Focus groups: A practical guide for applied research.* Newbury Park, California: Sage Publications.

Morgan, D.L. (1988). *Focus groups as qualitative research.* Newbury Park, California: Sage Publications.

Seidle, J.V., et al. (1988). *The ethnograph.* Amherst, Massachusetts: Qualis Research Associates.

Chapter 8

The Manager's Experience

Sue Luedtke and Barbara Haag-Heitman

You cannot teach a man anything. You can only help him discover it within himself.

—Galileo

MANAGEMENT COUNCIL ACCOUNTABILITIES

As the clinical practice development model (CPDM) transition was rolling out, the Management Council had several responsibilities, including the alignment of compensation to the nurses' level of skill acquisition as defined by the CPDM. Balancing the needs of the patients and skills of the nursing staff through examination and refinement of staffing patterns also needed to be addressed. Examining the institutional impediments to patient care identified in the narratives or through the peer review process was another important function of the management group.

Compensation Issues

Revision of the RN job descriptions was done to reflect the new expectations for clinical performance as defined in the CPDM. This included incorporation of the characteristics of practice into the text of the job descriptions as depicted in the Stage 3 (competent) job description in Exhibit 8-1. Working in collaboration with Human Resources, we moved from four job levels to five, which also necessitated revision in the pay scales. The current minimum and maximum pay scales were maintained while we stratified pay ranges within each stage. This task was easily accomplished because of the understanding the Human Resource Department had of the CPDM through their participation on the Steering Committee.

Exhibit 8-1 Excerpts from Stage 3 (Competent) Job Description

St. Luke's Medical Center
Milwaukee, Wisconsin

POSITION: Clinical Practice Nurse   DATE: April 1993
             Stage 3

POSITION PURPOSE:
The Clinical Practice Nurse Stage 3 is a professional nurse who performs the nursing process to deliver safe, therapeutic, quality patient care through assessment, planning, implementation, and evaluation.

REPORTING RELATIONSHIP:
Reports to Supervisor/Manager, who in turn reports to the Director/Vice President.
No subordinates formally report to this position, but the incumbent may give work direction to other ancillary nursing personnel.

ESSENTIAL FUNCTIONS:
Must demonstrate the characteristics of practice associated with the Clinical Practice Development Model Stage 3:

A. DEFINITION: Stage 3 competent nurses integrate theoretical knowledge with clinical experience in the care of patients and families. Care is delivered utilizing a deliberative, systematic approach, and practice is guided by increasing awareness of patterns of patient responses in recurrent situations. These nurses demonstrate mastery of most technical skills and begin to view clinical situations from a patient and family focus.

continues

Exhibit 8-1 continued

B. <u>**CHARACTERISTICS OF PRACTICE**</u>:

1. Clinical Knowledge & Decision-Making

    a. Demonstrates confidence in delivering Standards of Care.

    b. Provides care based on conscious, deliberate planning.

    c. Understands the expected progression of clinical events based on concrete past experiences.

    d. Desires to limit the unexpected by managing the environment.

    e. Assumes an increasing responsibility to advocate for patients and families.

2. Collaboration

    a. Recognizes their role and function as a member of the health care team.

    b. Delegates to other care givers as a means to help manage the clinical situation.

3. Caring

    a. Individualizes care and recognizes the personhood of patient and family.

    b. Are learning to establish and practice within the boundaries of therapeutic relationships.

Performs other duties as assigned or as necessity dictates.

Must meet the 'Performance Standards for Patient Care and Professional Accountability' as defined by the "Annual Performance Review Tool for Professional Nurses."

The Clinical Practice RN 3 must be able to demonstrate knowledge and skills necessary to provide care appropriate to the age of the patients served. The individual must demonstrate knowledge of the principles of growth and development over the life span and possess the ability to assess data reflective of the patient's status and interpret the appropriate information needed to identify each patient's requirements relative to his/her age-specific needs, and to provide the care needed as described in the department's policies and procedures. Age-specific information is developed further in the departmental job standards appropriate to the individual Clinical Practice RN 3.

Must adhere to established Service Standards.

Source: Courtesy of St. Luke's Medical Center, Milwaukee, Wisconsin.

Staff Utilization

We were challenged to rethink our usual patterns of staff utilization and balance the patient assignments and caseloads with the knowledge and capabilities of the staff nurses as revealed through the CPDM developmental stages. The CPDM convincingly illustrated the differences in practice know-how and helped shape our expectations for performance at each of the five stages. This heightened awareness influenced the process utilized by managers in making decisions regarding staffing, as noted in the following description by one of our managers:

> As a manager I have worked with many of the staff for most of their nursing career, but could honestly say that until the CPDM I never experienced the power of their exquisite practice. The narratives allowed me to understand and experience the staff nurse's practice in a way that was not possible before. I could see and feel the practice through the reading of the personal stories written through the nurse's eyes and heart. The CPDM process was extremely beneficial to both the CNS and me to assist in identifying the strengths and growth areas in each nurse's practice, which in turn helped us to plan strategies that would facilitate their growth. Knowing each nurse's developmental stage also assisted us in making staffing and hiring decisions to maximize patient outcomes. For example, by knowing our staff's developmental stages we could determine if we have the right mix of nurses to meet the needs of the patients that day.
> Courtesy of Joan Maro, RN

Use of the model in the hiring process is described by another manager.

> Using CPDM sets the stage as to the type of professional nurse we are looking for in our organization. In the interview process, when the CPDM is described and discussed as a condition of employment, many applicants view it very favorably and have commented that they feel they would be "in control" of their own professional growth using this developmental model with a peer review component. As a manager, the CPDM affords me the opportunity to recruit RNs who are self-directed and able to fully contribute to the outcomes needed for quality patient care and the success of our organization.
> Courtesy of Sue Katz, RN

Defining the unit mix of staff according to the developmental stages assists the nurse manager in determining the type of nursing skill needed to facilitate quality, cost-effective patient outcomes. Hiring decisions were facilitated with this knowledge. For example, if a general medical/surgical unit had mostly expert and proficient nurses, it would be reasonable to hire new graduates and advanced beginners. The more experienced staff would contribute to the care of the patients by collaborating with the newer nurses and overseeing the coordination of the care and assessment of the patient's progress toward the identified outcomes. They would also provide the mentoring needed to stimulate professional development of the new staff.

Another example of the usefulness of the model comes from the Family Practice Center, which is associated with a Family Practice resident teaching program. They were planning a change in the nursing care delivery model to better meet the needs of their patient population. At the time, they had a staff mix of RNs, LPNs, and medical assistants. Because of the complexity of many of their patients and families, there was need to coordinate care beyond the episodic clinic visit into the community and essentially along the entire care continuum. Their goal was to move to an RN case manager role and maximize the contribution of each of the other roles to accomplish the nursing plan of care. The leadership examined the skills needed to manage the complexity of this new work and found those qualities inherent in the characteristics of practice for expert and proficient nurses, several of whom were already on staff. As a result of this learning, it was decided to limit their hiring of additional RNs during this transition to those who were at the expert and proficient stages.

Redefining Relationships

As the process of transition unfolded, the true value of the CPDM began to emerge. From the manager's perspective, it was the opportunity to witness and publicly recognize the essence of professional nursing practice as told through the nurses' stories. Two nurse managers describe the importance of this relationship.

Knowing the practice on my unit through the reading of the staff's narratives keeps me connected to the practice in a profoundly significant way.

Courtesy of Mary Schigoda, RN

The greatest reward of management today is connecting with staff and the practice by reading the narratives and through the coaching experience. We often miss seeing all the wonderful things staff do for patients while we are concentrating on operational issues and planning for the future.

Courtesy of Judy Ploski, RN

The coaching component of the process opened up dialogue around the professional practice that had not been the modus operandi to this point. Managers, along with their clinical nurse specialist partners, now had a means to know the practice of all the staff on their units. As a result, individual developmental plans, specific to the stage and needs of the nurse, could be developed.

New knowledge of nurses' strengths and interests was also uncovered. For example, one of the operating room (OR) nurses wrote about her caring practices with patients who were in her area because they were experiencing miscarriages. She was very astute at identifying the patients' vulnerabilities and providing expert supportive care during very brief encounters in the OR. This unit had recognized that care of patients in the OR who were experiencing pregnancy loss was an area where enhancement was desired. Through her narrative, the ideal person to develop into the role of perinatal grief adviser for the OR was discovered. Each unit found its own hidden treasures in the narratives, such as nurses who had developed expertise in working with pain, domestic violence, and care of the dying.

The CPDM also helped the managers recognize vulnerabilities of nurses, particularly those at the lower stages of skill development. We discovered that the nurses on orientation thrived on the feedback and supportive role they received from their preceptors: "My preceptor helped me get through the code and talk with the family. She told me I did a good job." After orientation the need continued, but the supportive role of peers was not as present. As a result, we found the staff finding this recognition from the patient and family: "The patient said I was the best nurse they ever had." From our discovery of the importance of more frequent feedback to the staff in the year or so of practice following formal orientation, we made feedback from the experienced staff, manager, and the CNS a daily priority.

The model offered management an opportunity to become integrally involved with the clinical practice and staff in new ways. The importance of caring about our staff and the care they provide is unequivocal. Caring and trusting relationships were developed in the process. Recognizing and celebrating the extraordinary work of nursing has brought about a heightened sense of pride and has fostered the self-esteem of many of the staff. We have perceived that those staffs who feel good about their work and valued as employees are more fully engaged in the work. The effect on quality patient care can only be positive.

Recognizing our past history of "eating our young," the CPDM has been an excellent tool to demonstrate the natural progression of all nurses along the developmental continuum of novice to expert. Many of our experienced nurses have become much more supportive of the issues and concerns that show up for less experienced staff through the reading of their narratives. Understanding each other's contributions helps build a stronger team to meet the needs of the patients. The positive influence that the CPDM had on one manager's practice is described in the following account.

> I have found the CPDM to be enriching, enlightening, and a wonderful guide and support in my role as a manager and leader. Its research base is both logical and engaging. As I have gained experience with the model I have attained much insight and found it to be a beneficial professional tool that clearly articulates and identifies progressive behaviors. In my management role, the CPDM enhances my ability to appropriately delegate resources and anticipate certain outcomes based on where the nurse has staged along the developmental continuum. The CPDM assists me from a coaching and mentoring standpoint when there are issues regarding a nurse's perfor-

mance, as the model provides the language to discuss and hold staff accountable for their behaviors.

Professionally and personally I have grown as a result of my involvement with the CPDM. I have done additional study related to the novice-to-expert theory and application to the discipline of nursing from the human resource aspect of performance in my pursuit of an advanced degree in business management.

From that viewpoint I believe there is opportunity to refine the model to include more citizenship performance expectations.

Courtesy of Anne Meyer, RN

REMOVING SYSTEM BARRIERS TO PRACTICE

Since the implementation of CPDM, we have identified a variety of barriers to the provision of quality patient care. We have taken corrective actions to remove these impediments that may not have been revealed without the narrative methodology. One of the early recurring themes that emerged was that of staff struggling to obtain appropriate and timely physician responses during the night shift. Managers supported the staff to develop strategies to alleviate the problem, which included the creation of an algorithm to guide staff in solving these dilemmas when they occurred. Another system issue was uncovered in the narrative of an OR nurse working the night shift. She was called in to work in the middle of the night. During the case she went to the family waiting area to update the family on the patient's condition. While there, she received a page to call the OR. As she went to the phone to respond to the page, she discovered that the handset for the phone had been removed. Apparently there had been some thefts of the phones previously. She was unable to locate a phone in the area and needed to return to the unit, which was two floors away, to obtain the message. As a result of this story, the need to have working phones accessible to families and staff was illustrated and the phones are now in place in those areas.

Patterns of recurrent clinical incidents, which by themselves often seem isolated to the staff, have also been recognized. Reappearing stories of breast-feeding difficulties, epidural headaches, and difficulties scheduling patients for procedures came from a variety of staff, giving managers valuable data for corrective action plans.

POSTTRANSITION: USING KNOWLEDGE OF STAFF'S DEVELOPMENTAL STAGES TO ACHIEVE ORGANIZATIONAL GOALS

Managers, in partnership with other leaders in the entire organization, are continually challenged to respond to the increasing numbers and types of influences on our health care system. The need to align with the market demands for high quality and reasonable costs, along with the influence of the new emphasis of the Joint Commission on Accreditation of Healthcare Organizations (the Joint Commission) on the multidisciplinary focus on patient care design, compelled us to evaluate and redefine the staff nurse role. In collaboration with the Nursing Practice Council, we moved toward a new role component for the staff nurse as coordinator of care to continue to meet these demands.

The essence of the coordinator role lies in the principles of case management, centering on the organizing and sequencing of services to respond to an individual's health needs. Essential components for support of case management are similar to those of the nursing process and include health assessment, planning, and providing care in a coordinated effort along the health care continuum. Positive effects on cost, quality, and a decreased fragmentation of care can be realized as a result.

Our new knowledge of the staffs' practice from the CPDM afforded us the opportunity to develop the expert and proficient nurses into the new role of care coordinator. Specific descriptions from the CPDM (see Appendix C) define the strengths of their practice, particularly in collaboration and coordination that would support their transition to the new role component. These strengths are depicted in the CPDM definitions of the two roles:

Expert nurses collaborate with other caregivers to challenge and coordinate institutional resources to maximize advocacy for patient and family care in achieving the most effective outcomes. They value the expertise of the team members and creatively coordinate resources to provide the highest quality care for patients and families. Expert nurses influence practice by challenging the system and expanding boundaries to best meet the patient and family needs. They negotiate conflict by focusing on patient outcomes and promoting collaboration.

Proficient nurses develop effective relationships with other caregivers and provide leadership within the health care team to formulate integrated approaches to care. They mobilize other health care team members to achieve best possible patient outcomes. Proficient nurses recognize conflict and involve themselves to pursue the best patient outcomes.

Since over 75 percent of our staff nurses were staged at the expert and proficient stages, the development of these nurses into the care coordinator role was deemed a practical one. A specific and separate role of case manager was therefore not needed. These nurses continued to function as staff nurses with the addition of this new role expectation.

A PRACTICAL APPROACH TO ACHIEVING DESIRED OUTCOMES

The infrastructure for an effective design for care coordination was established through the collaborative efforts of the management, clinical nurse specialists, and the staff (Schifalacqua & George, 1999). A unit-based structure, referred to as Outcome Facilitation Teams (OFTs), was created. The teams are grounded in the principles of case management and use the expert and proficient staff nurses as the coordinators of patient care. These nurses facilitate the collaboration of other members of the health care team to efficiently accomplish defined patient outcomes. The nursing roles of unit-based nursing team on the OFTs are:

- Staff Nurse as care coordinator
- Manager as system linker and coach
- CNS as facilitator and mentor for practice issues and critical thinking skills.

Other disciplines that make up the core of the OFTs include social work, pharmacy, dietary, home care, and pastoral care.

OFTs meet five days a week to address individual needs of patients. The two key questions the team addresses are; "What is keeping the patient here today?" and "What are we doing to meet patient outcomes?" Documentation of all planned interventions is placed in the patient record.

It is the accountability of the manager and clinical nurse specialist to coach and facilitate this process daily. They focus on identifying and eliminating any real or potential system problems related to patient care. Since their implementation in 1996, the OFTs have demonstrated an increase in patient satisfaction, decrease in the length of stay, and an overall level of satisfaction from the providers. Managers find that allocation of staff mix according to the CPDM developmental stage can be more easily accomplished. The beneficial results for all the disciplines include:

- An increase in collaboration in care planning
- More timely and appropriate initiation of referrals
- Concerns of the family addressed earlier
- Discharge planning that truly begins on admission
- An outcomes/goals focus recognizable by all disciplines

Having a deep understanding of the practice from the narratives and the CPDM moved our organization away from developing another separate RN role as case manager at the unit level. Rather, the knowledge and skill of the bedside nurses are recognized and utilized in new ways. This change has been very satisfying to both staff and leaders in the organization.

SUMMARY

The new alliance developed with staff through the CPDM process, together with the new accountabilities and partnership defined in the shared governance model, laid the groundwork for shared decision making and autonomous practice, necessary for today's workplace. The power and possibilities of the CPDM are epitomized in this Chinese proverb:

If you want one year of prosperity, grow grain.
If you want ten years of prosperity, grow trees.
If you want one hundred years of prosperity, grow people.

REFERENCE

Schifalacqua, M.R., & George, V.M. (1999). The changing environment for outcomes management. Chapter 18 in Cohen, E. & DeBack, V. (Eds.), The outcomes mandate case management in healthcare today. St. Louis, MO: Mosby, pp. 162–170.

Chapter 9

Moving Beyond Transition: Enhancing the Process through Performance Improvement Activities

Theresa Dirienzo

Integrity without knowledge is weak and useless,
and knowledge without integrity is dangerous
and dreadful.

—Samuel Jackson

During the transition of over 700 staff nurses into the clinical practice development model (CPDM), most of the accountabilities for structuring and guiding the CPDM process resided with the Nursing Quality Improvement Council. With this enormous feat accomplished and the demand for promotional panels substantially decreased, attention turned to assuring the continuing integrity and quality of the process. This council was also undergoing transition; reflected in their name change to the Nursing Performance Improvement Council (NPIC) was the change in focus to performance improvement activities.

CPDM issues became a major focal point for much of the work done by the NPIC during the first years of its implementation. In response to our early learnings during transition, the applicant interview and coaching requirements had already been put into place. To assure clarity and integrity in all the essential components of the staging process, a comprehensive

Staging/Advancement Policy for CPDM was developed by the NPIC and is illustrated in Appendix D. This policy defined the staging time frames and criteria for initial and advancement staging; principles for the composition and writing of narratives; guidelines for panel membership and scheduling; and specified the role accountabilities for the applicant, coach, manager, facilitator, and panel members. The NPIC's accountability for approval of CPDM staging and advancement policy decisions was clarified in this document.

The integrity and quality of the CPDM process is continually monitored by the NPIC. Processes and accountabilities are well defined for all stakeholders in the CPDM Policy. Feedback mechanisms were created to monitor the quality of the entire process and respond to issues on a timely basis with corrective actions when indicated. Process improvements based on the feedback are discussed in this chapter.

Following the first two years of the CPDM implementation, St. Luke's Medical Center acquired a small local hospital, now named St. Luke's South Shore. Because this was an acquisition, it was necessary to transition an additional 80-some nurses into CPDM. The NPIC led the consolidation for CPDM, guided by the policies and procedures already set into place to again assure a quality process. The timeline for transition was again short because of other organizational issues. Calling upon lessons learned through our experiences during transition at SLMC, we relied heavily on the support of our experienced coaches from within the system to operationalize and support this change. A key learning from this experience was the confirmation of the validity of the application of the CPDM to another practice site, as evidenced in the feedback from South Shore applicants and their coaches, as well as an appeal rate of less than 1 percent. Both applicants and coaches remarked that the CPDM description of the practice had a goodness of fit to the practice setting as well. Interested South Shore staff moved into being active panel members for the peer review process with the same ease as did the St. Luke's staff.

TRANSITION PROCESS ENHANCEMENTS

Modifications to the CPDM policy occurred over time in the form of corrective actions based on issues brought to the attention of NPIC. The first major change, occurring during the transition process, was in the policy related to applicant interviews. A review of the application forms indicated that 50 percent of applicants were requesting interviews at the time of the panel review. Assessment of the peer review panel process indicated that the panel members were requesting interviews with the applicants an additional 25 percent of the time. This meant that 75 percent of applicants were already participating in an interview process. Initial interview times ranged from 20 to approximately 60 minutes. When considering whether to incorporate the interview as a mandatory component of the process, the council weighed the additional amount of time required to complete the panel process with an interview against the potential benefits of the interview. Recognized benefits to mandated interviews included immediate feedback to the applicant of the recommended stage and the ability to share and celebrate the nurse's contribution to patient care. Increasing panel member skill in the identification of characteristics of practice in the narratives, as well as experience in conducting interviews, suggested that a maximum of 30 minutes would be an adequate amount of time for the interview. To create consistency in the process, the interview was added as a mandatory part of the process.

Another early enhancement centered around coaching, which was also optional initially. Data indicated that 50 percent of applicants had utilized a coach, which, according to feedback from applicants and panel members, made the paneling experience more comfortable and easier for them both. Coaching seemed to facilitate a positive impact and a more productive panel interview. Since the goals of CPDM were to support and develop excellent practice, success, not failure, was to be encouraged. Coaching increased this possibility. The NPIC affirmed that coaching provided this support for the applicant and fostered the development of an ongoing relationship to identify strategies for continued clinical growth. The NPIC therefore stipulated that a coach be utilized by all nurses.

THE STARTING POINT: APPLICANT ACCOUNTABILITIES

Advancement along the novice to expert continuum is the accountability of each individual nurse with support from the organization's leadership. To begin the process, the applicant meets with his or her manager and CNS to discuss staging plans and determine whether he or she meets advancement criteria. When the applicant requests advancement and is determined to be eligible, the manager signs the application form verifying that the criteria has been met and the applicant may proceed with the process. Following or during the writing of three narratives, the nurse seeks out a coach and arranges for one-on-one coaching sessions to discuss the characteristics of practice identified in the narratives and how they relate to the CPDM framework. Chapter 6 describes further this learning relationship. As part of the process, the applicant does self-discovery of her or his developmental stage. It is the sole responsibility of the applicant to declare the CPDM stage being applied for. The applicant verifies that all of the processes related to coaching and the narratives are in place by signing the application form. The coach's signature on the application form signifies that the one-on-one coaching experience occurred and, to the best of the coach's knowledge, the clinical situations reported reflect the applicant's current clinical practice.

MONITORING THE QUALITY OF THE PEER REVIEW PANEL PROCESS

Skill development and qualifications of Peer Review Panel members are described in Chapter 5. Building and maintaining a skilled pool of panel members requires dedication by the participants. Panel members sign an agreement annually that signifies their willingness to meet the requirements and expectations as members of the panel pool. Role expectations for the panel member include commitment to participate in panels at least once every month. They further agree to come prepared to the panel having thoroughly reviewed the narratives. This review includes identifying the developmental stage along with the characteristics of practice and drafting interview questions that will enhance the understanding of the story. Maintaining confidentiality and promoting an atmosphere of trust and respect, thereby providing a positive experience for the applicant, are also required. The facilitator of the panel promotes the panel process by keeping the panel members focused on the characteristics of practice and interview discussion related to the CPDM framework.

One of the methods the NPIC uses to monitor the quality of the CPDM process is through the use of feedback forms given to the applicants and the coaches upon completion of staging (see Appendices E and F). The data are aggregated on a quarterly basis and analyzed by the council to determine whether concerns and trends are identified that require corrective actions and/or improvements. The current feedback forms have been utilized since December 1996. The importance of their feedback and use of the data is explained to the applicant by the panel. Applicants are given the option to complete the form prior to leaving after the interview, or taking the form with them to return in a preaddressed envelope to place in the hospital interoffice mail. All information provided via the feedback form is considered to be confidential.

Through analysis of the applicant and coach feedback data, the council is able to monitor the quality of the process and maintain the veracity of the model. The applicant feedback data continues to support the coaching experience as valuable in assisting the applicant to clarify the CPDM framework, prepare for the interview process, and establish a relationship by which strategies are identified for continued clinical growth. This data also provides ongoing evidence for the positive impact of the interview, which enhances the applicant's knowledge and understanding of CPDM.

The NPIC also reviews the many comments provided along with the feedback forms. Here are examples of statements made by nurses upon completion of the process:

- I have a good understanding of the CPDM process, which was supported by the panel. I wasn't surprised by any aspect.
- Panel members were very pleasant. I was nervous going in; however, the interview was very nonthreatening.
- I left my interview feeling very good about my practice. The interviewers reaffirmed my values as a nurse and helped me realize I am a good nurse.
- It helped me to understand this process by experiencing the interview. It was encouraging for me to hear experienced nurses give me feedback on my practice. It makes me feel like continuing with this process and striving for increased growth.

Obviously, along with the positive comments are the constructive criticisms, as revealed here:

- Writing of my narratives was the hardest thing, but my CNS and manager helped make writing them okay. My perception of staging was an awful one, but the help of CNS and manager and a great panel made it a wonderful experience.
- My coaching experience didn't start off on a positive note, but with the help of my manager, who assisted and encouraged me, it turned out okay.

The majority of the comments are supportive of the process. The NPIC does monitor the criticisms and suggestions provided by the applicants for trends that may require corrective actions. Data from the feedback received is presented to the nursing staff at the Professional Nursing Assembly meetings, which are held every other month. Data directly related to the coaching role is processed with the CNS department due to the high percentage of this group in the coaching role.

MONITORING PANEL OUTCOMES

There are four possible outcomes following the panel staging process. Applicants can be staged (1) at the level applied for; (2) lower than applied for; (3) higher than applied for; or (4) not staged, as the panel could not reach consensus. In addition, the applicant can appeal the decision and seek the opinion of a second panel. Table 9–1 presents the staging results during transition and over the next 3 years. Over 75 percent of applicants have achieved their applied-for stage over the years, reflecting the effectiveness of the coaching relationship, thoughtful self-reflection by the applicants, and skill of the panel members. Acquirement of a stage higher or lower than requested has remained stable for the most part, aside from a slight increase noted in year 2.

APPEALS

An applicant has the option to appeal to a second panel. This might occur when a candidate's panel staging recommendation is a stage lower than the applicant applied for. The appeal application must occur within 30 days of the NPIC confirmation of the initial panel's stage recommendation. The applicant is required to submit the same three narratives reviewed originally by the first panel. The facilitator of the second panel is aware that this is an appeal panel. The members of the second

Table 9–1 Outcomes from Staging

Time period	Number of nurses	At request stage %	Lower than requested stage %	Higher than requested stage %	Appeals %
Transition	711	76	19	5	2
Remainder of Year	22	96	4	ø	ø
Year 2	98	88	6	5	ø
Year 3	185	82	12	6	<1
Year 4	204	76	10	11	<1

panel are informed of the appeal status just after consensus discussion of CPDM narrative characteristics and interview questions are determined. There is no communication between the first panel members and second panel members. Specialist representation is present on all appeal panels. To decrease the anxiety for the applicant, appeal panels are scheduled as quickly as possible and they take priority for scheduling. After confirmation of staging from the second panel, documentation from both panels is reviewed by two validated NPIC designees to establish panel inter-rater reliability. The designees review for consistency in the identified characteristics of practice within the narratives, and for documentation of interview questions and resultant characteristics that are revealed through the interview process. A discussion with the two facilitators may be necessary to clarify their respective processes and to enhance growth of facilitation skills. A summary of these findings is then forwarded to NPIC.

The appeal rate has remained low, with only three appeals in the three years following transition. This low rate speaks to the reliability and validity of the model and quality of the process. The majority of appeals occurred during the transition phase of CPDM, when panel members, coaches, and applicants were learning and acquiring new skills.

PANEL OF NONCONSENSUS

There are rare circumstances when the panel members cannot agree on a recommended stage after the interview. The applicant is told that a recommendation cannot be made and that a second panel will review the original narratives. This can be a very difficult process for the applicant and the panel members, and another panel review is scheduled as quickly as possible.

The second panel has specialty nursing representation and the facilitator is the only panel member that is aware of the nonconsensus status from the first panel. The facilitator does not share this information with the panel members until after the applicant interview process is complete for the second panel.

During the CPDM transition, there were only two such panels from over 700 panels, which were promptly repaneled. Both subsequent panels were able to reach consensus and successfully stage the applicant.

ONGOING MONITORING OF THE PROCESS

Every month, the NPIC meets to confirm the staging recommendations made by the panel for nurses having completed the CPDM process. The council reviews each applicant's paperwork to ensure all components of the process are intact, as stated in the CPDM policy. Documentation to support the characteristics of practice for the recommended stage must be found within the narratives. The final written review from the panel resembles the documentation evidenced in the validation packets (see Chapter 5). The qualifications for the panel members and coaches is also evaluated. When the process is determined to be intact, the applicant's stage is confirmed by the council. If a break in the process has occurred, the NPIC applies the policy to interpret the action needed in individual circumstances. An example of a break in process was identified when a nurse failed to achieve the stage she applied for based on the lack of supportive characteristics for that stage identified in her written narratives. The applicant shared during her interview that her coaching experience was that of a one-time 10-minute phone conversation. The NPIC determined that this was not an adequate coaching experience and therefore the applicant's stage could not be confirmed. The council's decision was that the nurse would seek out a meaningful coaching experience as defined in the policy and reapply for staging once this had been accomplished. A few months later this nurse did successfully complete her staging.

Another example of a break in process occurred when, during the interview process with the panel, an applicant who had recently returned to work at the same facility after several years disclosed that all three of her narratives were from clinical experiences that took place prior to a leave of absence, approximately seven years ago. The CPDM policy states that narratives must be reflective of the individual's current practice and must be clinical experiences that have occurred in the past year. Upon discovering this information, the interview process was stopped, the CPDM policy reviewed with the applicant, and the NPIC chairperson as well as the applicant's coach were notified of the break in the process. The applicant did complete her staging process at a later date, utilizing patient experiences to illustrate her current nursing practice.

Occasionally quality of care and/or systems concerns have been revealed through either the narratives or the interview process. The NPIC addresses these concerns and directs corrective actions, which may include referrals, as needed, to individuals, units, or councils. One illustration of a quality-of-care concern surfaced through narratives for a specific unit. The nursing unit was experiencing barriers when attempting to contact physicians to deal with patients' problems. Continually, they were instructed by certain doctors to notify different physicians, which affected the timeliness of care provided to the patient. The unit's manager was informed of the concern and assumed the accountability for corrective action and monitoring of the issue.

The CPDM, as it prevails today, is the result of five years of dedication and determination to achieve a vision that recognizes and celebrates nursing practice at the patient's bedside. Nursing is a great deal more than the various technological functions often associated with the profession. Through narrative accounts of nurses' interactions with patients and families, a wonderful revelation of the richness of nurse/patient relationships has blossomed, contributing to positive clinical outcomes for the patient and family.

Chapter 10

Metro Clinical Practice Development Model: Redesign for the Region

Sharon Gray

You cannot step twice into the same river,
the waters are forever flowing by.

—Heraclitus

When the vision of a major health care corporation includes "regionalization" of services, all components of the organization begin to design the strategic plan necessary to meet the goal. Systems that were once separate undertake the task of collaborative unification. St. Luke's Medical Center (SLMC) is but one entity within the Metro Region of Aurora HealthCare. Four hospitals are included in the Metro Region:

- Hartford Memorial Hospital (HMH), Hartford, WI
- St. Luke's Medical Center (SLMC), Milwaukee, WI (includes St. Luke's South Shore)
- Sinai Samaritan Medical Center (SSMC), Milwaukee, WI
- West Allis Memorial Hospital (WAMH), West Allis, WI

In February 1998, these four hospitals began the work of creating a nursing clinical professional development model to be utilized across the region. This chapter describes the journey of the design team in achieving this mutual goal.

HISTORY

In 1997, Aurora HealthCare completed a major revision of its strategic plan. Subsequent to the completion of the system strategic plan, the regions within Aurora began the work to build strategic alignment across the system. System integration was a major goal, with the purpose of advancing Aurora as an integrated health system in which the system components functioned interdependently. Governance would be aligned to facilitate the advancement of an integrated delivery system. This would be accomplished by creating a regional governance body within the Aurora system governance structure. To this end, nursing began its integration process by designing a whole system shared governance model; specific to the discipline of nursing but with adaptability to a multidisciplinary model.

Within the context of nursing shared governance came the creation of the Metro Nursing Transition Steering Committee (MNTSC). The MNTSC was composed of nurse leaders from across the region and was dedicated to establishing the major themes of the strategic goals for nursing across the Metro region. The Steering Committee provided functional coordination of four decision-making subcouncils. In addition, the MNTSC created five transitional design teams to address major Metro initiatives. The design teams were nondecisional and would provide recommendations that the MNTSC would act upon. The work of all of these groups, including implementation and evaluation of initiatives, was coordinated through the MNTSC. Exhibit 10–1 defines the membership of the MNTSC. Exhibit 10–2 illustrates the structure of the MNTSC and its councils.

In the fall of 1997, the MNTSC, its subcouncils, and nurses across the Metro region met to determine the strategic plan. Among the major themes identified for strategic goals was the development of nursing accountabilities. The vision was articulated: "There will be an accountability-based practice model that guides RNs in the metro region and defines the unique contribution that the RN makes to the health of the community." The Metro Practice Council was charged with developing

Exhibit 10-1 Membership of the MNTSC

- Four (4) Staff Nurse Presidents/Chairs of Governance Systems (of the four regional hospitals)
- Four (4) Staff Nurse Chairpersons of the MNTSC Subcouncils
- Four (4) Staff Nurse Chairpersons of MNTSC Design Teams
- Chief Nurse Executive of the Metro Region
- Metro Region Director of Nursing Operations/Clinical Integration
- One (1) Director of Patient Care Services
- One (1) Patient Care Manager
- Manager of the Clinical Nurse Specialists

Source: Courtesy of Aurora HealthCare-Metro Region, Milwaukee, Wisconsin.

Exhibit 10-2 Structure of the MNTSC

- Coordinating Council, Metro Nursing Transition Steering Committee
- Subcouncils of the MNTSC (decisional)
  - Metro Education Council
  - Metro Leadership Council
  - Metro Performance Improvement Council
  - Metro Practice Council
- Design Teams of the MNTSC (nondecisional)
  - Metro Communication/Cultural Transitions Team
  - Metro Information Technology Design Team
  - Metro Professional Development Design Team
  - Metro Research Advisory and Design Team
  - Metro Shared Governance Design Team

Source: Courtesy of Aurora HealthCare-Metro Region, Milwaukee, Wisconsin.

a common nursing conceptual framework that incorporated care across the continuum.

The professional practice of nursing would be grounded in the conceptual framework. Within this domain, the need for the continuing professional development of nurses across the region was identified. The Metro Practice Council established goals for integrated system implementation in 1999. One of the strategies identified to meet this goal was the creation of a common professional development model. In February 1998, the MNTSC identified the need to create the Professional Development Model Design Team. The design team would report its recommendations to the MNTSC. The MNTSC would provide final approval for, and coordinate implementation of, the design team's recommendations.

THE DESIGN TEAM

The MNTSC appointed the chairperson of the design team. The chairperson was a clinical nurse specialist (CNS) from St. Luke's Medical Center, who had participated in the development of the Clinical Practice Development Model (CPDM) and remained involved in the process. This chairperson would provide design team liaison to the MNTSC. Membership on the design team would come from the four hospital entities within the region. All nurses on the design team would represent the profession of nursing and not specifically their entity. They would, however, serve as the communication linkage with their geographic locations and peer groups across the region. Membership of the design team included:

- CNS Chairperson
- 10 staff nurses
- one Director of Patient Care Services
- one patient care manager
- one CNS, in addition to the CNS Chairperson
- one Human Resources representative
- various consultants identified as experts who would be used on an ad hoc basis

A call for staff nurse membership was made. Staff nurses applied for the committee based on specific membership criteria. The criteria for membership and application content are shown in Exhibit 10–3. In March 1998, the MNTSC (with the involvement of the design team chairperson) reviewed the staff

Exhibit 10-3 Criteria and Application for Membership

Criteria for Membership

- Staff nurse at point of service
- Recognized as a strong clinical role model
- Strong leadership and communication skills

Application Content

- Demographic information: name, title, stage or level on current development model (if applicable), hospital and unit of origin, means of contacting
- Clinical experience and nursing background
- Applicant's reason for interest in the design team
- Applicant's anticipated contribution to the design team
- Description of previous experience with career ladder/ development model design

Source: Courtesy of Aurora HealthCare-Metro Region, Milwaukee, Wisconsin.

---

nurse applications and made the final selection for the design team. Every attempt was made to select members who would represent the widest range of clinical specialties, metro facilities, and experience with career ladders/developmental models. In order to create opportunities for broader participation across the region, the steering committee also tried to include members who were not currently involved in Metro leadership activities. The remaining members (those who were not staff nurses) of the design team were approached, based on experience and interest, and appointed by the MNTSC.

DESIGN TEAM CHARTER

The Professional Development Model Design Team met for the first time in April 1998. A draft of the team charter was discussed by the members and finalized at that meeting. The purpose of the design team was to (1) review the literature regarding annual performance review, career ladders, and professional development models, (2) differentiate advantages and disadvantages of each concept, and (3) explore actual models in operation at various health care sites.

The Professional Development Model Design Team was not a decision-making council. The team would be responsible to collaborate and communicate with the appropriate subcouncils of the MNTSC, specifically with the Metro Practice Council. The outcome of the team's activity would be to make recommendations to the MNTSC regarding a model that would be used by all staff nurses across the Metro region for clinical development, recognition, and advancement. The design team would also make recommendations regarding the design of the model and the implementation plan. The MNTSC would make the final decision and would direct implementation of the model.

The scope of the model was defined as including all staff nurses at point of service, in ambulatory and inpatient settings, at the four hospital entities within the Metro region. The hospitals in the region were very diverse, ranging from a community-based hospital with 120 nurses to an urban tertiary-care facility with more than a thousand nurses. Staff nurse performance evaluation tools varied widely among the entities. Issues were inequality in salaries, job codes, and merit adjustment. The new development model needed to provide:

- A process that would standardize the job codes, key functions, and salary ranges across the region.
- A systematic approach to converting staff from their current job code to a new Metro system (the annual performance review process occurs in April and triggers a merit adjustment. All nurses must be equitably assigned to an appropriate salary range).
- A common language to describe clinical nursing practice across the region.
- A consistent and reliable means of recognizing and advancing nurses as they develop.

CLINICAL FOCUS DETERMINED

All four hospital entities presented their current method of nursing performance evaluation. Members described what they perceived as the strengths and weaknesses of their evaluation tools. Once again, great diversity was identified. The only commonality between the four hospitals was that they all had annual performance evaluation (APR) in place. One hospital (SLMC) had a clinical practice development model. One hospital (SSMC) had a career ladder. The other two hospitals (WAMH and HMH) had no additional mechanism for staff nurse evaluation. Utilizing current literature on performance evaluation (both nursing and business) and the mechanism of group discussion, differences in the various approaches were defined, as noted in Exhibit 10–4.

Once this process had occurred, it became evident to the design team that consensus had been reached on several key points. The purpose of the group was again clarified: To design and recommend a professional development model that described clinical practice behavior expectations for RNs providing direct patient care. The model must maintain awareness of and be grounded in the conceptual framework of practice; therefore, as it did not address clinical practice, annual performance review (APR) would be eliminated from consideration. Since WAMH and HMH used only APR, their language would not be used in the development of the model. Both SSMC and SLMC included elements of clinical practice in their tools; these two tools would be utilized for future comparison in model design.

The model would include a consistent mechanism for advancement related to clinical performance, and would describe the accountabilities at different levels of practice. There would be a focus on the work of professional nurses at point of service, with universal accountability and expectations for nurses across the region. Citizenship issues would need to be addressed through the Human Resources annual performance evaluation.

Having decided on a model based on clinical practice behaviors, the group then moved on to discuss important elements the model would need to have. The list of the elements is identified in Exhibit 10–5. Nursing literature was consulted again, with a focus on clinical performance evaluation. The list of

Exhibit 10-4 Difference in Characteristics of Evaluation Tools

| Annual Performance Evaluation (Merit) | Recognition and Advancement | | Professional Development Model (Benner's Novice to Expert) |
	Career Ladder	
Predominately based on: • Nonclinical activities (i.e., committees, educational projects, charge role) • Good citizenship (i.e., attendance, teamwork, flexibility with hours) • Basic skills competencies	In addition may include: • Clinical activities and behaviors • Demonstrated by documentation of care (i.e., care plans) • More dialogue about clinical goals		Seven domains of clinical nursing practice: • Helping • Teaching/coaching • Diagnoses and monitoring • Management of rapidly changing situations • Administering and monitoring treatment • Ensuring quality • Organization and work roles
Quantitative measures of practice. Often a point system.	Quantitative measures of practice May include more consistent measures of competency. Correlated to levels within the framework.		Qualitative measures of practice. Analysis of specific characteristics of nursing practice: • revealed in narratives • correlating to stages of development within the framework

Inconsistent interpretation of criteria and merit. Weighted according to the values of individual managers.	More consistent criteria. May include some elements of peer review.	Research-based model. Reliable and valid analysis of practice through narratives. Coaching and peer review
Hierarchical: up and down movement of promotion and demotion	Hierarchical: up and down movement of promotion and demotion	Movement is one-directional progressively increasing development.
Externally motivated and acquired. Criteria according to the values the individual organization.	More internal motivation to participate or not.	Internally motivated to integrate knowledge and experience into clinical practice.
Manager is the gatekeeper of recognition and promotion.	Primarily manager-driven with some peer input.	Solely peer review related to staging/advancement.

Source: Courtesy of Aurora HealthCare-Metro Region, Milwaukee, Wisconsin.

important elements, and the SLMC and SSMC evaluation tools, would be compared to existing nursing literature.

BENNER'S NOVICE TO EXPERT MODEL IS CHOSEN

By the end of May 1998, members both familiar and unfamiliar with the concept of clinical performance evaluation came to the same conclusion. The design team reached consensus that the Benner novice-to-expert model of professional development came the closest to containing the important elements that were identified by the group. The design team decided to look exclusively at Benner and communicated this decision to the MNTSC.

Members of the design team were challenged to evaluate the Benner model in its entirety, and undertook the task of educating themselves specifically on the Benner theory, model of development, and methodology of clinical practice evaluation. Benner-specific literature was made available and an RN consultant was brought in to present the Benner model and theory. Experience with novice to expert at SLMC and other hospitals was discussed. Actual models (including CPDM) were distributed for the members to review and critique.

Reservations regarding the Benner model revolved around the use of narratives to illustrate the stage of clinical practice, and the process of peer paneling for staging. Would we simply use the novice to expert language (as had been done in the SSMC career ladder), or would we validate and utilize the entire process as described in the current CPDM model used at SLMC?

Anxiety around peer review concerned the ability of nurses to evaluate the narratives and stage their peers successfully. Would those who did not share a common area of practice with the applicant be able to evaluate the narratives accurately? Would they be able to recognize the elements of practice in an unfamiliar setting or at a different hospital?

Experience at SLMC validated the ability of the peer panel to utilize the model criteria and accurately stage the applicants, despite the various practice settings of the panel members. In addition, participants in the paneling process actually found it

Exhibit 10-5 Important Elements for Model Design

- Valid and reliable tool that equitably measures the practice it is intended to measure.
- Measures outcomes and is based on nursing behavioral language/practice.
- Peer review; no manager as "gatekeeper."
- Comprehensive in defining whole practice, and universal across settings and continuum of practice.
- Model reflects mission, vision, and values of Metro Region.
- Not cumbersome, easily understood, "user-friendly."
- Provides linkage to orientation and education.
- Philosophy impacts staffing pattern; patient assignment based on level of expertise.
- Includes "future visions" link to research and outcome facilitation.
- Flexible in evolving as health care nursing practice evolves.
- Core themes are represented across the stages of the model.
- Model assures continuous accountability. You "live it" and expectations are articulated in the model. Provides clarity of accountability.
- Behaviors across a continuum are reflected in the model.
- Model provides a celebration of practice and a way to be recognized (privilege/title/monetary)
- Ensures opportunities for both growth and mentorship.
- Growth behaviors are defined as a way to move along the model.
- There is a correlation between salary and advancement.
- There is a correlation between increased development and increased "opportunity."
- Applicable to nurses across the region.

Source: Courtesy of Aurora HealthCare-Metro Region, Milwaukee, Wisconsin.

to be a positive experience. Indeed, nursing practice was celebrated during the paneling process. Design team members recognized in advance that staff would articulate these concerns and decided to address them through education in the implementation phase.

The use of narratives as the evaluation mechanism engendered the most concern and discussion. The fears expressed were consistent with the concerns articulated in the original implementation of CPDM at SLMC. Staff nurses worried that the level of writing skill would influence their ability to stage high on the ladder. They expressed disbelief that practice could truly be evaluated through the mechanism of storytelling. The process of writing narratives itself caused stress:

- How would nurses be able to remember their stories?
- How would they find a story interesting enough to the panel members?
- What types of stories qualified for narrative writing?

The fears that centered around narrative writing were acknowledged, and the group began to examine narratives in order to educate themselves and to validate their use as the evaluation methodology.

Staff nurses on the design team were asked to write a narrative and there was a call for stories from staff nurses across the region. CNSs and patient care managers were asked to engage two or three nurses from their units in the writing of a clinical story. These same leadership people were also asked to write a clinical story from the perspective of their roles. This would give the leaders an opportunity to experience written storytelling and to develop empathy with the staff nurses as they began to engage in dialogue about their practice. Guidelines for composing clinical narratives were provided. Nurses were apprised of the design team's intention of incorporating the principles of Benner's novice-to-expert domains of practice into the new Metro model. Clinical behavior elements from the current tools at SSMC and SLMC would also be utilized. The design team would use the narratives in identifying characteristics of practice, with the goal of developing a common language to describe nursing across the region. They would also, hopefully, allay the fears described by the design team and realize the validity of the narrative methodology.

As the staff nursing narratives arrived, they were compared to the qualifying statements included in the clinical domains of the various stages of the Benner model (replicating the original process used at SLMC). Clinical practice across the region was indeed comprehensively reflected in the stories of the nurses. In addition, the sharing and discussion that took place brought about the realization that the narrative was a powerful and valuable means of articulating the contribution of nursing to health care.

> In my role as a resource nurse I assisted with the evaluation process at annual performance review. Every year I listened to RNs complain about the career ladder process used to measure their performance. Most felt the process was too subjective, redundant, and most importantly, didn't give enough credit and recognition for their clinical accomplishments. I applied to participate on the Metro Developmental Model Design Team hoping to assist with developing a model that would be satisfying and rewarding to the nurses.
>
> Initially the idea of writing narratives to describe nursing practice seemed inconceivable. I felt strongly that three stories describing a clinical situation could not adequately reflect all that a nurse does to facilitate patient outcomes.
>
> As I began to read actual narratives written by nurses within the organization, I was able to see the identified behaviors that described the various stages. "Believing" came when I began the process myself; writing my own narratives. I realized the narratives were revealing more about my individual practice than could ever be revealed by observation alone. I am left feeling that this exploration of ourselves will result in a far greater appreciation and understanding of what we do and how well we do it.
>
> Courtesy of Malea Rodziczak, RN, Staff Nurse
Sinai Samaritan Medical Center

> In March of 1998 I submitted my application to participate on the Aurora Metro Professional Development Model Design Team. I truly believed that nursing needed some form of recognition for their practice at the bedside other than the subjective Annual Performance Review. I had previously been involved in an unsuccessful career ladder program and wanted to have some input into a model that would affect my colleagues and me. I was determined NOT to get involved in a model that required narrative writing like another hospital in our region was already using to evaluate their practice. There *had* to be a better way!

I was chosen to participate on the design team. It was a hard-working group representing all facilities in the Metro region with both acute care and outpatient nurses. I vowed to myself to keep an open mind. We evaluated different theories and practice models and discussed ways these could be implemented. We weighed their pros and cons of each. As all the models were discussed we kept coming back to the Benner model. It made the most sense!

I also came to realize that narratives were the most honest and nonjudgmental way of describing practice. Combining narratives with peer review was the model of choice for us. I was "sold" and supportive of a practice model and process I swore I would never do.

Courtesy of Beth Horwath, RN, Staff Nurse
West Allis Memorial Hospital

Time and time again, the design team marveled at the ability of the stories to reveal the strength of holistic practice and the commitment to the well-being of the patient. Consensus was reached that the Metro developmental model would utilize the Benner novice-to-expert framework in its entirety. This recommendation was communicated to the MNTSC. In late June 1998, the MNTSC accepted this recommendation and defined the timeline and plan for implementation. All nurses across the region would be staged on the new model prior to annual performance review (and merit determination) in April 1999. Two subcouncils of the MNTSC were charged with responsibilities regarding the MCPDM. Refer to Exhibit 10–6 for the subcouncil accountabilities.

CREATING THE METRO CLINICAL PRACTICE DEVELOPMENT MODEL (MCPDM)

Resources needed for development of the model were collected and distributed to the design team members. See Exhibit 10–7 for a catalogue of resources. The team identified anxiety around the struggle to achieve the reality of the short timeline for implementation. Each team member described his or her current experience with the professional development model, rumors, staff concerns, and issues around implementation. Through this process, future direction for implementation was

Exhibit 10-6 MNTCS Subcouncil Accountabilities to MCPDM

Metro Practice Council

- Define practice across the region within the context of the Metro Conceptual Framework for Nursing
- Evaluate the MCPDM and accept it for use in the Metro Region

Metro Performance Improvement Council

- Define the process for MCPDM, including the policy and procedure
- Coordinate the development of all aspects of the MCPDM implementation
  - Staff education regarding Benner/MCPDM and narrative writing
  - Development of trained coaches and panel members
  - Implementation and monitoring of the staging process

Source: Courtesy of Aurora HealthCare-Metro Region, Milwaukee, Wisconsin.

determined. Consensus was reached and members committed to the support of the shared governance decisions of the MNTSC.

The purpose of the narratives solicited from across the region was twofold: (1) to identify characteristics of practice and validate the current model, and (2) to explore the opportunity for additional characteristics and domains within the model.

SLMC evaluated the CPDM in 1995, and had identified the desire to add a domain that centered around teaching in the nursing role. Reviewers of the proposed change had determined there were not enough descriptors to support the creation of an entirely new domain, therefore, these recommendations had never been incorporated into the model. The current design team process was the first extensive reevaluation of the original model and the group wanted to insure that the current state of practice was reflected in the new model. In addition to reinvestigating the teaching domain, the design team had identified the need to include the component of research in the model.

Exhibit 10-7 Catalogue of Resources Used in Model Design

- Benner texts and related literature
- CPDM currently in use at SLMC
- Career ladder currently in use at SSMC
- Benner feedback on the CPDM process at SLMC
- SLMC suggestions for revision to the current CPDM
- Benner-based developmental model frameworks from other organizations
- Metro Philosophy of Nursing and Conceptual Framework drafts
- Narratives from all entities
- Narratives from Benner Internet web site

Source: Courtesy of Aurora HealthCare-Metro Region, Milwaukee, Wisconsin.

Work began by focusing on identifying the characteristics of the Expert at stage 5 of the model. Characteristics of the current models under investigation were assigned to the clinical domains of Coordination and Collaboration, Clinical Knowledge and Decision-Making, and Caring. The Metro Research Council was consulted and assisted the team in defining the research criteria for practice in each stage of the model. The new research statements were included in the Clinical Knowledge and Decision Making domain. Education was investigated as a new domain. It was discovered in the process that the domain of "teaching" was much broader than patient and family teaching. The domain was expanded to include the subcategory of Professional Development and Self-Learning. The statements for research and for the new domain of Education are shown, for the Expert level, in Exhibit 10–8.

Every stage of the model was designed using the regional narratives for validation. New narratives arrived from staff almost daily and were incorporated into the process along the way. Once the design team had completed the first draft of the model, it was shared with those staff nurses who were currently serving as panel members in the CPDM. The panel members were those nurses who had the most experience with "living"

Exhibit 10-8 Research and Education at the Expert Level

I. Research

Collaborates with other caregivers to challenge current practices and synthesize research findings to develop optimal systems to achieve the most effective patient and family outcomes.

II. Education (a new domain)

  A. Teaching Patient/Family

    1. Maximizes utilization of resources to meet patient/family learning needs.

    2. Assists the patient/family to incorporate condition-related issues into lifestyle changes.

    3. Accurately assesses and uses the patient/family's readiness to learn to promote patient teaching at a time that is suitable.

    4. Modifies the situation or environment to create the teachable moment.

    5. Anticipates learning needs and creates a plan proactively.

    6. Manages clinical demands of situations while encouraging patients/families to participate in care and decision-making.

  B. Professional Development and Self Learning

    1. Critically evaluates own decision-making and judgments, and engages in professional development activities to increase the quality of these decisions.

    2. Recognizes knowledge of self to maintain objectivity and separate personal feelings within ethical/moral situations.

    3. Portrays a professional image and positively influences practice.

Source: Courtesy of Aurora HealthCare-Metro Region, Milwaukee, Wisconsin.

---

the model and could articulate any difficulties in using CPDM. The panel members provided valuable feedback, proposing thoughtful and eloquent ideas that were used to refine the model. The model was completed in August 1998.

IMPLEMENTATION

All nurses who delivered direct patient care would be staged on the MCPDM prior to Annual Performance Review in April 1999. Nurses at SLMC would be exempt from restaging during transition, as they had already been staged on a comparable model. Every effort was made to ensure the process would be as "user-friendly" as possible, with the focus on education and facilitation of the individual nurse's progress.

In July 1998, Dr. Richard Benner of Benner Associates arrived to provide consultation to the design group and education on the Benner model to the staff and nursing leadership. A presentation, in which Dr. Benner described the novice-to-expert theory and the validity of narratives, was scheduled for all CNS's and patient care managers. The leadership team was pivotal to the successful implementation of MCPDM and must be able to articulate and support the reasons for choosing the model.

Following the presentation to nursing leadership, Dr. Benner traveled the Metro Region to present the model to the staff nurses. Presentations were scheduled over two days for each entity (HMH, WAMH, and SSMC), with one presentation at SLMC. As many staff nurses as possible were encouraged to attend. A powerful component of the presentations was the reading of a narrative by a staff nurse on the design team. In order to assist in making the process "real" for the staff attending, the nurse reading the narrative was from the entity in which the presentation took place. The presentation by Dr. Benner was followed by a question-and-answer period mediated by nurses from the individual hospitals and by nurses with CPDM experience. Staff nurses voiced the fears that had been anticipated by the team, most centering around questioning the need for change and the process of writing narratives.

Following the Benner presentations, timelines for implementation were distributed. Timelines were designed for the staff nurse who had to stage, the staff nurse who desired to be a panel member, and managers and CNS's who would be utilized as coaches to the staff nurses. Sample timelines for staff staging and coaching validation are shown in Exhibit 10–9. There was a

Exhibit 10-9 Sample Timelines: Staging and Coaching

Staff Nurse Staging	Coaching Validation
Attend Benner presentation (7-98)	Attend Benner Presentation (7-98)
View Benner videotape	View Benner Videotape
Begin to write narratives	Attend coaching class by 8-15-98
Attend narrative writing class (9-98)	Begin to attend coaching sessions as co-coach
Schedule coaching session (9-98)	Complete and submit coaching validation packet by 9-1-98
Complete narratives and submit for staging by 10-15-98	Begin to observe paneling process as "silent fourth" member
Await scheduling of panel staging	Receive validation as coach
Complete panel process and staging by 12-31-98	Begin coaching staff by 9-15-98

Source: Courtesy of Aurora HealthCare-Metro Region, Milwaukee, Wisconsin.

wealth of knowledge and experience at SLMC in the form of panel members, and CNS and manager coaches. The nursing leadership at SLMC were designated as mentors and facilitators to the process, and each nursing leader was assigned to a specific area in one of the hospitals that needed to stage.

In the original staging of CPDM at SLMC, the benefit of coaching was recognized early on for its positive impact on the staging process and identification of specific developmental strategies for each nurse. Based on these experiences, similar implementation strategies were utilized for the Metro transition.

At the time of publication, transition to the Metro Clinical Practice Development Model was proceeding smoothly. The clamor that accompanies any major organizational change had been minimized by the excellent efforts in education and mentoring. The staff nurse was beginning to recognize the value of the MCPDM process in validating and "growing" practice.

Planned evaluation of the process will address the need for revision and will enhance the evolution of nursing practice in the Metro Region of Aurora HealthCare.

Chapter 11

Future Trends: Advancing Professional Practice in an Interdisciplinary Model

Carol Camooso

The rung of a ladder was never meant to rest upon, but only to hold a man's foot long enough to enable him to put the other somewhat higher.

—Thomas Henry Huxley

As we prepare to enter the next millenium, trends are emerging that will impact the way nurses and other health care professionals provide care. The drivers underlying these trends are demographics, technology, and funding. With an increasingly aging population, emphasis will shift to chronic diseases such as heart disease and cancer (Girvin, 1998). The focus of health care organizations will shift from treating illness to health promotion; from care focused on the individual to community and population-focused care. Emphasis will shift from acute care to care along the continuum of prevention, early intervention, acute care, and chronic long-term care (England, 1997). Readily accessible information will result in more educated consumers (Grayson, 1998). Growth in technology will improve clinical outcomes and will influence the knowledge, skills, and attitudes required by health care providers. Alternative therapies will become complementary therapies. The portion of patient care funded by the government will increase, and, with movement to capitation and prepayment, economic risk will shift from the government and employers to health plans, providers, and consumers (Grayson, 1998; Fubini, 1997). Purchasers will establish long-term contractual relationships with organizations based on the "value" of care (cost/quality) rather than based on cost alone (England, 1997).

There is some debate among health care pundits and policy makers, however, regarding which organizational designs will best promote the delivery of efficient, high-quality services at moderate costs. Many believe that vertically integrated networks supported by databases will be the best means to provide "seamless care." Opponents believe that integrated networks attempting to provide "everything to everybody" will be difficult to sustain over time; they advocate for organizations focused on providing a range of services for patients with a specific, chronic disease or disability diagnosed in the primary care system (Herzlinger, 1998). Though this debate may continue into the twenty-first century, it is now recognized that clinicians' ability to collaborate in an interdisciplinary way will be the key to an organization's effectiveness in meeting the challenges and demands of the future.

It is within this context that Massachusetts General Hospital (MGH) nurses and other health professionals are implementing strategies that enhance quality, strengthen our position in the current competitive market, and establish a foundation for the future. This work is being done within the framework of the MGH mission, which is *to provide the highest quality care to individuals and to the community, to advance care through excellence in biomedical research, and to educate future academic and practice leaders of the health care professions.* Health professionals continue to collaborate to provide personalized, highly skilled care. They also add to the body of knowledge and to advancements within their respective disciplines. These advancements continue as MGH transforms itself with an eye on the future. MGH, not unlike other organizations, is forming new strategic alliances with other area hospitals; primary care physicians and specialists are forming networks to capture increasing shares of the health care market. Leadership is capturing the creativity of employees in a process to redesign operational systems to increase efficiency. They are challenging health care providers across disciplines to define different and better ways to deliver care while maintaining professional values.

In order to enhance the environment in which this dialogue can occur, MGH leaders have also realigned the reporting relationships of the various departments. One of the significant administrative changes has been the alignment of clinical departments under a senior vice president for Patient Care. This administrator, who is a nurse, is also the chief nurse executive. The departments include Nursing, Respiratory Therapy, Occupational Therapy, Speech-Language Pathology, Physical Therapy, Social Services, and the Chaplaincy. There are concerns described in the professional literature that nurses, in a structure such as this, fear they will lose autonomy and position; other disciplines may feel that a nurse will not understand their practice and issues (Lockwood, 1995). Contrarily, the MGH experience has been that it has been facilitative to have health care providers that are organized around the patient be organized around the administrative table as well. This structure minimizes departmental barriers and promotes an environment for shared decision making and problem solving. This interdisciplinary redesign has also established the foundation for other initiatives that have supported professional empowerment and have enhanced communication, planning, and shared learning among the disciplines in Patient Care Services. These major interdisciplinary initiatives include *articulation of a professional practice model* and *implementation of a collaborative governance model*.

INTERDISCIPLINARY PROFESSIONAL PRACTICE MODEL

Our actions to prepare for the future are framed by our patient-focused vision, core values, and guiding principles (Figure 11–1). It emphasizes that our primary focus is the patient and recognizes the importance of the relationship

Figure 11–1 Patient Care Services Vision, Values, Guiding Principles

Our Vision

As nurses, health professionals, and Patient Care Services support staff, our every action is guided by knowledge, enabled by skill, and motivated by compassion. Patients are our primary focus, and the way we deliver care reflects that focus every day.

We believe in creating a practice environment that has no barriers, that is built on a spirit of inquiry, and reflects a culturally competent workforce supportive of the patient-focused values of this institution.

It is through our professional practice model that we make our vision a demonstrable truth every day by letting our thoughts, decisions, and actions be guided by our values. As clinicians, we ensure that our practice is caring, innovative, scientific, and empowering; and that it is based on a foundation of leadership and entrepreneurial teamwork.

Our Values

Our core values include:

- Excellence
- Integrity
- Compassion
- Leadership
- Patient Focus
- Diversity
- Innovation
- Scholarship
- Accountability and responsibility
- Responsiveness and decisiveness
- Entrepreneurial teamwork
- Cost and resource effectiveness

Our Guiding Principles

- We are ever-alert for opportunities to improve patient care; we provide care based on the latest **research** findings
- We recognize the importance of **encouraging patients and families to participate** in the decisions affecting their care.
- We are most effective as a team; we continually strengthen our relationships with each other and actively promote **diversity** within our staff.
- We enhance patient care and the systems supporting that care as we work with others; we eagerly enter new **partnerships** with people inside and outside of the Massachusetts General Hospital.
- We never lose sight of the needs and expectations of our patients and their families as we make clinical decisions based on the most **effective use of internal and external resources.**
- We view **learning as a lifelong process** essential to the growth and development of clinicians striving to deliver quality patient care.
- We acknowledge that maintaining the **highest standards of patient care delivery** is a never-ending process that involves the patient, family, nurse, all healthcare providers, and the community at large.

Our vision, values, and guiding principles are intrinsically linked to our commitment to provide the highest quality, culturally competent care to our patients and their families.

Source: Courtesy of Massachusetts General Hospital, Boston, Massachusetts.

Figure 11–2 Patient Care Services' Professional Practice Model

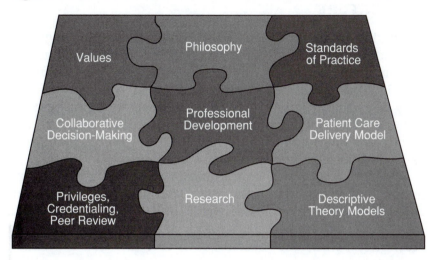

Driven by a commitment to provide the highest quality care to patients and their families, every element of the model "interlocks" to ensure the delivery of seamless, knowledge-based patient care.

Source: Courtesy of Massachusetts General Hospital, Boston, Massachusetts.

between clinician and patient and family. The vision is grounded in the understanding of the rich contributions that each of the professional disciplines and support staff bring to relationships with patients, families, and the interdisciplinary team as a whole (Ives Erickson, 1996).

Guided by this vision, Patient Care Services launched an interdisciplinary professional practice model. Represented by an "interlocking" puzzle, each "piece" of the model represents a component of practice (Figure 11–2). Each component is related to all of the others. Together, these components bring depth to our practice. Development within each of these components brings nurses, physical therapists, occupational therapists, respiratory therapists, speech-language pathologists, social workers, and chaplains the knowledge and skill needed to enhance practice.

INTERDISCIPLINARY COLLABORATIVE GOVERNANCE STRUCTURE

Building on a shared vision and professional practice model, Patient Care Services initiated an interdisciplinary collaborative governance structure in June 1997. Just as the administrative redesign has facilitated communication among interdisciplinary department heads, collaborative governance has created the infrastructure to promote communication among caregivers. The MGH collaborative governance structure comprises eight committees, five of which are interdisciplinary (Exhibit 11–1). This model is a communication and decision-making model that places the authority, responsibility, and accountability for patient care with the practicing clinician (AONE, 1996). Collaborative governance is built on the premise of "teamness"; clinicians come together to create and implement

Exhibit 11–1 Patient Care Services Collaborative Governance Committees

Interdisciplinary Committees:	
• Quality	The focus of the Quality Committee is to review clinical quality issues with an eye toward identifying opportunities for integrating quality initiatives into clinical practice.
• Professional Development	The Professional Development Committee is charged with designing a clinical recognition program for clinicians within Patient Care Services. Work includes defining program objectives, recommending implementation strategies, and identifying criteria for program evaluation.

continues

Exhibit 11–1 continued

- Ethics in Clinical Practice — The Ethics in Clinical Practice Committee was formed to develop and implement activities and programs to help further clinicians' understanding of the ethical aspects of patient care. The work of this committee involves identifying strategies to integrate judgement into professional practice.

- Patient Education — The Patient Education Committee's work involves developing processes for patient and family education, recommending systems and technology to support improved patient education, and ensuring that all materials and activities reflect the diversity of populations we serve.

- Patient Care Services Diversity Steering — The Diversity Steering Committee is dedicated to developing strategies that support diversification of the workforce within Patient Care Services in order to meet the diverse needs of the patients we serve. The work of this committee includes professional development, student outreach, programs centered around culturally competent care, and input into the development of patient-education materials for use by clinicians with diverse patient populations.

Nursing Committees

- Department of Nursing Practice — The focus of the Nursing Practice Committee is to review, revise, and communicate standards of practice

continues

Exhibit 11–1 continued

	for professional nursing at the MGH. Their work includes reviewing and approving new products and new practice recommendations, and communication outcomes and revisions to staff throughout Patient Care Services.
• Nursing Research	The Nursing Research Committee exists to foster a spirit of inquiry around clinical practice. The committee supports nurses in the research process, communicates the results of institutional research activities, and reviews research proposals related to nursing policy, procedures, and Institutional Review Board (IRB) requirements.
• Staff Nurse Advisory	The purpose of the Staff Nurse Advisory Committee is to provide a forum for communication between nursing leadership and clinical nurses at the MGH. Committee members representing all patient care units dialogue with nursing leaders about matters of patient care and professional development.

Source: Courtesy of Massachusetts General Hospital, Boston, Massachusetts.

actions toward a desired outcome. Through participation in the committees, clinicians from various disciplines have been able to readily interact with one another, present different perspectives about patient care, expand their awareness of hospital initiatives, broaden their knowledge base, and enhance their ability to make decisions. It is an infrastructure through which those around the patient have been able to work together to innovate and advance patient care and professional development (Ives Erickson, 1997).

PROFESSIONAL DEVELOPMENT COMMITTEE

Ongoing professional development is a strategy for successfully preparing clinicians for changes occurring in health care. The Professional Development Committee was convened in July 1997 to create a professional development and clinical recognition program for clinicians within Patient Care Services. The committee leadership includes two staff co-chairs (a registered nurse and a therapist) and a leadership coach who is a nurse who assists members with agenda setting, group process, and project support. Membership, which currently numbers 22, is composed primarily of direct-care providers; one member is a nurse manager and one a therapy director. The variation in the numbers of representatives from each discipline reflects the variation in the size of the respective departments. Most members are registered nurses representing unit types based on patient population. There is one representative from each of the therapies and social service. The committee meets twice a month for two hours.

It is clear that the major challenge is to develop a professional development and recognition model that is interdisciplinary, one that can provide a generic framework across the disciplines, yet highlight the uniqueness of each profession. Currently, there are differences among the disciplines regarding the types of programs already in place. Three of the therapy departments have advancement programs with positions at the advanced level limited by the budgeted number. One therapy department, social service, and nursing have no formal programs. In addition, at the time members began its work, there were differences regarding which aspects of professional practice should be recognized. Should an advancement program focus on clinical practice only, or should it include aspects of practice such as committee work and level of education? Discussion about educational preparation was complicated by the differences among the disciplines regarding entry level education. Nursing has multiple entry levels compared with Social Services and Speech Language Pathology, which require a master's degree as a minimal level of education. This variation among the membership and the disciplines made this project initially daunting.

The galvanizing force among the membership was their agreement, early on, that they needed first to articulate the themes of practice within the disciplines as the foundation of any professional development and advancement program. Members identified clinical narrative review as the methodology through which this would occur. They also adopted the Dreyfus model of skill acquisition as the framework they would use to describe the developmental levels of clinicians. This was based on the assumption that the Dreyfus model, applied to the work of nursing by Patricia Benner, could be applied to other disciplines as well. Committee objectives for the first year included collecting and analyzing narratives to describe themes of practice and educating our multidisciplinary staff and leadership about the Dreyfus model of skill acquisition and the clinical narrative methodology. The senior vice president for Patient Care engaged a consultant to assist the committee in its work.

ARTICULATING THEMES OF PRACTICE THROUGH CLINICAL NARRATIVES

At the time the decision was made to use the clinical narrative methodology, there were varying levels of awareness throughout the disciplines regarding narratives. The use of clinical narratives has a fairly long history in nursing at MGH. Patricia Benner and MGH nurses have had many dialogues about the nature of clinical practice as reflected through our narratives. In 1996, the senior vice president for Patient Care initiated the regular inclusion of clinical narratives into our biweekly hospital publication as a way to make visible the knowledge embedded in practice. It is through this mechanism that many of the health professionals became aware of storytelling as a way to share practice. Narratives submitted for publication reflected primarily situations about which the clinician felt they made a difference. Authors received assistance as needed to ensure clarity and readability of the story.

When the committee introduced narratives as the means to describe practice, the goal was to have uncoached narratives from skilled clinicians throughout various patient care areas and departments in Patient Care Services. It was unclear how many narratives would be sufficient to reflect practice. With guidance from the consultant, members believed two narratives from each nursing unit would ensure that the narratives would reflect nursing practice provided in all areas. However, it was unclear how many narratives would be required of the therapists and social workers. The numbers of clinicians varied within these disciplines, ranging from 17 speech-language pathologists to 57 respiratory therapists. Initially, members specified a 10 percent sample and requested two to five narratives from the therapies and social service, depending on the department size. After further consideration, however, members believed this small number might not be sufficient to capture the themes of the discipline. They decided to continue to collect narratives within these disciplines until no new themes emerge.

The committee designed and implemented a process to collect narratives. This was achieved through obtaining names of "skilled" clinicians from each Nurse Manager and Director. There was no attempt to define "skilled." These clinicians received letters from the committee co-chairs indicating that they had been identified as a skilled clinician and requesting that they submit a clinical narrative to the committee for review. The letter emphasized that the review would be anonymous in order to avoid bias during the review process and promote openness by the author. In order to increase comfort with the narrative process, support materials regarding how to write a narrative were enclosed with the letter. The materials included tips on writing a narrative and provided samples. It clarified that clinicians could choose to write stories about one of several types of clinical situations that held meaning for them: situations where they felt their interventions really made a difference; situations where things went unusually well; situations where there was breakdown; situations that they feel described the essence of their practice. Initially, there was a moderate response to the committee's request. In part, this was due to "myths" about the clinical narratives, somewhat related to the high quality of those which appeared in the Patient Care Services publication. Clinicians misperceived a demand for excellent writing skills, assumed that situations about which they wrote needed to be extraordinary, and feared that the narrative had to be lengthy. These and other myths were somewhat dispelled through discussion by the committee coach with staff individually and in groups and by addressing the myths in the Patient Care Services publication.

REVIEW PROCESS FOR THEMES OF PRACTICE

There was discussion regarding whether there should be interdisciplinary analysis of narratives or whether each discipline should review and analyze their own. It was unclear whether the themes that emerged would differ among the disciplines. Ultimately, members initiated an interdisciplinary review process, primarily to grow together in the ability to review and interpret information in the narratives. At this time, it also became clear that, to complete the work within an acceptable time frame, it would be necessary to add a second monthly two-hour meeting. Because not all members could make this commitment, the second meeting was composed of all the therapy and social service representatives and a subset of the nursing members. The subgroup meeting was dedicated to review of the narratives. The second hour of the full committee was also limited to narrative review in order to facilitate the review work getting done and to ensure that all members would share the experience of and become comfortable with narrative analysis.

Initial discussion about the process for review included whether members should review the narratives using an organizing framework such as the domains described by Benner (1984). The group considered whether Benner's domains would be applicable across the disciplines and began the review process by having the members read the narratives together and identify relevant themes. After two or three weeks of review, it was evident that an organizing framework would facilitate the process, and Benner's domains were used. The group concurred, over time, that Benner's domains were applicable across disciplines, though they emerged differently and perhaps with varying frequency among the disciplines. For example, managing rapidly changing situations emerged more frequently in nursing and respiratory therapy narratives than in physical therapy narratives.

As review continued, there appeared to be differences in the nature of the storytelling among the disciplines. Nurses' stories seemed to focus more frequently on the helping role, particularly around end-of-life issues; therapeutic interventions were frequently present, but as a backdrop rather than the main point of the story. It was not uncommon for nursing narratives to describe situations that were unresolved for the nurse. In contrast, narratives by the therapists were rich in descriptions of the therapeutic interventions they individualized for patients. The differences in the narratives may reflect the differences in the nature of the disciplines. It may also be explained by the frequency with which some of the therapies use case study as a developmental tool. This awareness led to discussion regarding differences between the case-study approach and the narrative approach. Members agreed that while both described the assessment and interventions, narratives could provide a more complete picture of the ethical and psychosocial complexities of care as well as more fully describe what the clinician was feeling and thinking during the clinical situation. The consultant suggested that those who wished could start with a case-study approach and build on it.

Interdisciplinary review and discussions in such areas as those described above ultimately resulted in an increased appreciation of the theoretical underpinnings of practice among the disciplines, much more so than members had anticipated. Even though clinicians worked side by side with the patient, interdisciplinary review provided the opportunity for clinicians to describe to those in other disciplines the subtleties of the practice reflected in the narrative. Interestingly, as the narrative review proceeded, three major themes emerged consistently across the disciplines: clinical knowledge, clinician-patient relationship, and teamwork and collaboration. What follow are clinical narratives by a speech-language pathologist, a nurse, and a respiratory therapist, which illustrate the presence of these themes.

Speech-Language Pathologist

In this narrative, the speech-language pathologist describes a situation in which her involvement made a significant difference in the outcomes for a 43-year-old, previously healthy female who had suffered a massive pontine cerebellar stroke. This patient was presumably "locked in" (unable to communicate verbally and unable to move her arms and hands to assist with communication). Through skilled application of her clinical knowledge and her ability to presence herself with this patient, she assisted the physicians and nurses in empowering this patient to make decisions about her care.

> This last May I was approached by a resident and several nurses alerting me about a patient who needed assistance in communicating her wishes and an immediate assessment to determine her ability to comprehend.
>
> Mrs. H's volitional motor movements were limited to up-down gaze and partial lateral with the left eye. It was most important to everyone on the team (especially for the nurses, who showed great compassion for this patient) to determine if she could understand and communicate in order to empower her to make her own decisions regarding her care. Major issues such as tracheostomy, G-tube, and prognosis needed to be addressed. Everyone felt that the patient, if she could, should make these decisions.
>
> As I read the medical record, many thoughts crossed my mind. "I have a tremendous responsibility here. If this were me, what would I do?" I remembered another locked-in patient I had seen years earlier, who, despite my spending hours with him week after week, never was able to communicate with others. I knew that my role now was to obtain objective data in a systematic way, but only sharp observational skills and quick thinking were going to help in this situation.
>
> It was 2:00 PM when I went in to see her. She was intubated and appeared comfortable. I observed her for at least 15 minutes. She was not aware that I was in the room. I observed all of her reflexive movements so that I would not misinterpret involuntary movements for volitional responses to my questions. There was a sign on the

wall, "Up gaze—Yes, Down gaze—No." I introduced myself and immediately sat down on a stool to achieve eye contact. She was so young, not much older than I was. I explained who I was and my purpose. I was sure that if she indeed understood what I was saying, she must have experienced some hope of finally being able to ask questions and express thoughts. I knew the reality had changed. For someone like her to be able to express complex thoughts, modern electronic equipment was going to be required, none of which I had.

I had a very structured plan which began with yes-or-no questions, progressed to reading words, and finally to an alphabet board. Although my assessment plan was complex and systematic, it was a gut feeling that helped me move from one task to another in order to maintain her attention and the rapport that was initially established. At times I slowed down or sped up, other times I reminded her of the purpose of our session, and twice we just talked.

I had objective data to prove that she could process auditory and written information and could choose answers to specific questions via written words. Implementation of a system in which the patient could generate her own words still remained a hope.

After accurately identifying letters through a tedious but specific approach, I asked her to spell a word related to a thought she had. You can imagine what a challenge that is when you only have the ability to gaze up and down. After selecting first rows and then specific letters, she spelled the word BREATH. She wanted more information about the endotracheal tube and the vent. She also communicated the word PROGNOSIS. I realized that she was indeed locked in. The exercise soon fatigued her and I knew I had to leave, but at least I had some answers for the team.

On May 13, with two family members present, Ms. H. indicated that she wanted a tracheostomy.

Registered Nurse

In this narrative, the nurse describes two experiences that were particularly meaningful to her in her care of a 22-year-old college student who was admitted to the bone marrow transplant unit. In the telling of this story, the themes of clinician-patient relationship and collaboration strongly emerge as she helps grant this patient one of her last wishes and presences herself with this patient in discussing end of life-issues.

"A" was a senior college student and was diagnosed with leukemia. This was quite a shock to her because she was only sick with a "bad cold" for two weeks. When she went to the infirmatory [sic], they drew some blood and discovered her nightmare—she had leukemia. "A" initially went to another major hospital to be treated, but her leukemia did not go into remission despite three attempts of chemotherapy. She was then referred to us for a "last chance effort."

When I met "A", there was a real connection between us. She was very bright and articulate. She was very easy to work with each day. We enjoyed each other's company and had some common interests. I was amazed as to how she dealt "head on" with her disease and treatment. She wrote in her journal every day and would sign each entry with "IWSL". This meant "I will survive leukemia."

There were many experiences I shared with "A." But there are two experiences that are special to me. The first was the day "A" wanted to take a tub bath. "A" was very sick that day—she was neutropenic, she had terrible mouth sores, her strength was minimal, and she was on numerous IV antibiotics and drugs. She required a great deal of assistance from the nurses. Her only wish that day was to sit in a "nice hot tub bath." This was not going to be easy. First of all, where could I find a tub she could use, and second, how would I get her in and out of the tub without any problems. But my instinct told me to try my best to give her this wish. I knew this would be one of her last wishes.

I called over to the labor and delivery unit - They told me there was an empty room with a Jacuzzi tub bath that "A" could use. "A" was so excited! Along with her mom, I took "A" to the other unit. The tub was filled with wonderful, warm water. With the assistance of her mom, we guided "A" into the tub. She was so delighted. "A" had the biggest smile. She said the bath was "absolutely glorious". She sat in the tub for about 1 hour. She thanked me a thousand times that day. This was very satisfying to me and I knew I had made a big difference in her care.

The second experience I shared with "A" is when she was told that the treatment was not working and that she was going to die. This was one of the most difficult but heartfelt experiences in my career. After she was told by the bone marrow team (including myself), "A" was devastated. She didn't want to speak to anyone after she was told. I told her when she was ready to talk about it, to let me know. Just as I was about to leave at the end of the shift, her mom came to get me and told me that "A" wanted to talk to me now.

I went into "A's" room—just the two of us. Through her tears, we talked for over an hour. She asked me questions. One of the questions was, "What would you do if it was you?" She desperately needed help to make this decision. Should she "give up" and go home with hospice? We talked about how it wasn't fair for a 22 year old girl, what it was like to die, what it would be like in heaven, how she would be an angel and she also felt she could take care of people after her death.

"A" also asked me to give her the entire syringe of morphine. She said, "Let's get it over with now! Please do it!". I told her I would not give her the entire syringe of morphine. But I would keep her comfortable and help her with any questions. I would be there for her.

I have never been asked by a patient before to "get it over with." This request was very distressing to me, but certainly portrays "A's" strength and courage.

The next day, "A" decided to go home with hospice. I went to visit her at home. The minute I saw her in her room, surrounded by her family, and the cat curled up on her bed, I knew she had made the right decision. She looked very comfortable and peaceful. She was so happy to see me and was very thankful for all of my help. "A" died five days later, surrounded by all of the things she cherished.

Respiratory Therapist

This clinical situation describes this therapist's collaboration with team members as she tries to optimize the respiratory status of an infant. Clearly recognized by others as skilled clinician, she effectively applies her clinical knowledge and promotes a sense of peer support.

Recently, I was working in the Pediatric Intensive Care Unit (PICU). The morning had been busy, but by mid-day things were relatively quiet. I knew my colleague was having a busier day in the Neonatal Intensive Care Unit (NICU) so I went over to see if she needed any help. When I walked into the unit, I was greeted by one of the NICU attendings. He asked if I would look at a patient who was not doing well to see if I had any recommendations for managing the infant's respiratory care. He gave me a brief report on a 24-week gestational age infant, now three months old, who had just recently been transferred to MGH for a surgical procedure. The baby had been difficult to oxygenate and required ventilator support since birth but was now requiring 100 percent oxygen and becoming more difficult to ventilate. The latest blood gas demonstrated severe ventilatory failure with a marginally acceptable oxygen level despite receiving 100 percent oxygen.

I was immediately interested in seeing if I could help the infant, but I thought it best not to just jump in. I decided first to talk with my colleague working in the unit. When I approached her, I remarked that Dr. X had mentioned there was a baby who was difficult to manage. Her response made me aware that she and others had already tried different approaches to ventilating the infant but nothing seemed to matter. I listened as she said "We should just leave the kid alone. It doesn't matter what we do. His lungs are a mess." I sensed her frustration but thought that from the information she had given me that not all possible approaches to his management had been exhausted. I told her I was not sure if I have anything to offer the baby, but asked if she would want to take a look at him together. She agreed.

Approaching the bedside, I spoke with the nurse to let her know I was just taking a look as I had been told the baby was having a difficult time. She too expressed frustration at how poorly the kiddo was doing and talked of the difficulties associated with caring for him and his parents. With one look at the infant, I was immediately struck at how hard he was working to breathe. My first question was, "Does he always work this hard?" His respiratory rate was 112, he was retracting, had an active expiratory phase, his oxygen saturations were in the 80s, and his heart rate was an active 160–175. Both the therapist and the nurse agreed that this was "baseline" since arrival at MGH. I gathered a little more information from the nurse and therapist and decided to adjust several parameters on the ventilator. I explained to the therapist what my rationale was for each of the moves. Within minutes, the infant's respiratory rate, heart rate, and work of breathing had all improved. The oxygen was weaned from 100% to 75%.

The attending physician came to the bedside and I explained to him the approach we had taken. Everyone agreed the infant had not looked this comfortable since arrival. Together we established a plan. As long as the infant continued to appear more comfortable, we would leave him on the new settings, wait 30 minutes, then check a blood gas. I then returned to the PICU to continue working with the patients I was assigned.

About two hours later my colleague came over and told me the baby still looked good, the blood gases were significantly better, the parents were in and were thrilled with the infant's improvement. Now, could I come over and look at another patient.

The consistency in themes reflected in these narratives reflects the true application of a shared vision for patient care. It also exemplifies that care is not provided in isolation within a discipline but is practiced in an interdisciplinary environment where care is influenced by the shared values within the organization. Narratives had accomplished the goal of discovering and describing practice.

CLINICAL NARRATIVES AS TOOLS TO ENHANCE PROFESSIONAL DEVELOPMENT

In addition to the consultants providing guidance to committee members with narrative analysis, they also provided interdisciplinary educational forums for clinicians and leadership. These were one- and two-day sessions that included forums for all role groups. Topic areas included Dreyfus model of skill acquisition, application to nursing by Patricia Benner, and elements to be considered in implementing advancement programs. There were many sessions during which authors read their narratives and the consultant demonstrated coaching techniques. These sessions led to a heightened awareness of the power of clinical narrative methodology in enhancing professional development. The use of narratives as a means to describe themes of practice within the Professional Development Committee has expanded to a highly effective method for clinicians to reflect on and grow their practice. This provided the rationale for continued integration of narrative methodology as a professional tool for clinicians in Patient Care Services.

CONTINUING STEPS

Currently, the committee work to describe practice through narrative analysis is occurring in parallel with the work of Patient Care Services' departments to expand the use of clinical narratives as a developmental tool.

Within the Committee

- Members are expanding narrative analysis to define behaviors at three developmental levels (beginner/advanced beginner, competent, and expert), using the themes of clinician-patient relationship, clinical knowledge, and teamwork and collaboration as a framework. This activity is being done by clinicians within each discipline with the guidance and assistance of their committee representative and committee coach.
- Members, in collaboration with the senior vice president for Patient Care, are beginning to define strategies to describe a recognition/advancement program in Patient Care Services. The goal is to identify a program that can be integrated into the programs already in place within disciplines.
- Meetings of the complete committee membership have increased from once to twice a month; the narrative review subgroup has been disbanded. This change will increase the regular involvement of all members in narrative review.

Within Patient Care Services

- The Professional Development Committee and the senior vice president for Patient Care will continue to require narratives as part of the professional portfolios submitted by nominees for The Expertise in Clinical Practice Award. The purpose of the semiannual award is to recognize the expert application of values reflected in our vision.
- Nurse Managers, Directors, and clinical leadership in Patient Care Services' disciplines are expanding the use of clinical narratives as a way to promote self-reflection and encourage professional development. Two Professional Development Coordinators from the Department of Nursing's Center for Clinical and Professional Development are assisting them in helping clinicians write and review clinical narratives. Included are strategies to increase the comfort level of those who will assume the coaching role.

SUMMARY

In this chapter, the author described the evolution of an interdisciplinary administrative model, a shared professional practice model, and an integrated collaborative governance structure. Within this framework, clinicians applied the Dreyfus model of skill acquisition and clinical narrative methodology as a strategy to promote a shared understanding and language of practice and professional development while highlighting the unique contributions of each discipline.

This work is being done within a context of a rapidly changing health care environment in which we must meet the challenges of today while preparing for the future. Professional literature warns of "turf wars" that may be fought among health care professionals, with nursing at the center. It cautions about the potential for skills being reduced to technical tasks among unlicensed personnel, and professional boundaries becoming blurred and identities lost among the professionals (Gottlieb, 1997). The interdisciplinary framework and approaches described above make visible the knowledge embedded in practice and highlight the uniqueness of the professions. Fostering an environment in which individualized, holistic care is provided, it is also setting the stage for effective, interdisciplinary work, which will be key to successful organizations of the future.

REFERENCES

AONE Leadership Series. (1996). *The business of nursing.* Chicago: American Hospital Publishing.

Benner, P. (1984). *From novice to expert.* Menlo Park, CA: Addison Wesley.

England, M. (1997). The evolving healthcare system: Changing paradigms and the organized systems of care. *Journal of Allied Health, 27*(1), 7–12.

Fubini, S. (1997). A collective vision of healthcare in the year 2020. *Nutrition, 13*(1), 62–63.

Girvin, J. (1998). Future imperfect: A conference. Healthcare—the next millenium. Nursing Management (London): *Nursing Standard Journal for Nurse Leaders, 4*(8), 8–9.

Gottlieb, L. (1997). "Co-opetition": A model for multidisciplinary practice. *Canadian Journal of Nursing Research, 29*(1), 3–5.

Grayson, M. (1998). An interview with Dick Davidson. *Hospitals and Health Networks*, July 5, 12–16.

Herzlinger R. (1998). The managerial revolution in the US healthcare sector: lessons from the US economy. *Health Care Management Review, 23*(3), 19–29.

Ives Erickson, J. (1996). Our professional practice model. MGH *Patient Care Services Caring Headlines, 2*(23), 1–2.

Ives Erickson, J. (1997). Collaborative governance is here! *MGH Patient Care Services Caring Headlines, 3*(12), 1–2, 14.

Lockwood, B. (1995). Developing the role of vice president of Patient Care Services: Pulling the clinical team together. *Recruitment, Retention, & Restructuring Report, 8*(7), 4–7.

Chapter 12

Defining the Essence of Health Care Practice through Novice to Expert Models: Research-Basis and Future Opportunities

Laura J. Burke and Marie P. Farrell

Research without practice is folly, but practice without research is blind.

Benner (1984) used qualitative research to examine the knowledge embedded in narratives of clinical nursing practice. From these narratives, she described a novice to expert model of acquiring skills in nursing. We replicated the Benner approach at St. Luke's Medical Center and created a Clinical Practice Developmental Model (CPDM) for nursing (Haag-Heitman and Kramer, 1998; Ladewig, Haag, and Webber, 1994; Nuccio et al., 1996). Subsequently, we expanded the model for nursing as the Aurora HealthCare Metro Clinical Practice Developmental Model (MCPDM). As a measure of validation, we reviewed other institution's novice to expert models. For example, a team at Massachusetts General Hospital in Boston, Massachusetts developed the Interdisciplinary Professional Practice Model (IPPM). These models, based in California, Wisconsin, and Massachusetts, when contrasted with one another, appear to provide representations of clinical nursing practice or interdisciplinary health care practices.

The purpose of this chapter is to describe the processes model developers used to ensure that the models are valid, reliable, and meet the criteria expected of models that represent the practice of direct patient care. We raised the questions that our organizations challenged us to answer and we described the steps we took to develop a refined set of research questions. The ultimate aim was to define the elements essential in delivering nursing and health care to ensure quality at the bedside.

ARE NOVICE TO EXPERT MODELS VALID AND RELIABLE?

When novice to expert models were implemented in the three above-mentioned hospital settings, the staff at each hospital asked: "How do we know the models are valid?" That is, "How do we know a particular model will truly represent our practice?" Also they asked, "How do we know that the process of applying a model is reliable?" That is, "How do we know that different groups of staff would come to the same conclusion based on the same set of evidence?"

Administrative and human resources staff raised the same questions of reliability, but posed a different question about validity: "How do we know that the staff's narratives are valid?" That is, "How do we know that these narratives truly represent the staff's current practice?" These questions underscore the need to examine the issues of rigor surrounding the models' development and their application.

The staff in the organizations evolved specific strategies to strengthen the models and the rigor of the application processes. We summarize these strategies here and discuss the implications of applying these models for research and clinical nursing practice.

INTERNAL VALIDITY, CREDIBILITY, AND AUTHENTICITY

In qualitative research, internal validity is sometimes referred to as credibility (Miles and Huberman, 1994) and addresses the question, "Do the models authentically represent the experience as described by the participants?" The participants, in this case, were the health care providers who delivered direct patient care and documented their care through their written narratives. During the design of the models, the teams used the same strategies to assure that the models truly represented their disciplines as practiced.

First, the participants worked to ensure that the universe of the discipline's practice (e.g., nursing, physical therapy, dietetics, etc.) were represented in the narratives by using specific sampling strategies to generate narratives from a variety of practitioners. For example, at St. Luke's Medical Center, staff from 93 percent of the inpatient and ambulatory nursing areas contributed to the pool of narratives used to create the CPDM. When staff at Massachusetts General Hospital conducted a similar exercise, they used a minimum sample of narratives from 10 percent of their staff in each discipline. Ultimately, they gathered a sufficient number of narratives to reach "theoretical data saturation" to create the IPPM. Theoretical data saturation is a process of collecting data until a sense of closure is attained because new data yield only redundant information (Polit and Hungler, 1995).

Second, to guard against biased data collection and to minimize acquiescent responses, staff purposely were not coached. That is, they were asked to "simply write narratives or exemplars that described a key learning moment in their practice." The team gave minimal direction to lessen the likelihood that the narrators would write to meet expectations rather than to describe their clinical practice. Lastly, the teams used member checks, debriefing, consensus building, and negative case analysis to guard against biased data interpretation. Specifically, the teams used large committees comprised of staff who represented those who would use the model. The committee members independently reviewed the narratives and made notes describing key behaviors such as, "evaluates the patient/family's understanding of teaching provided" or "negotiates conflict by focusing on patient outcomes and promoting collaboration." Members debriefed each other by building consensus concerning the language they used in the models. The teams also conducted negative case analyses to identify areas where data did not fit with the emerging theoretical framework. Because the members of the committees were staff, member checks were an inherent component of the consensus building process.

The teams used specific strategies during the implementation of the models as clinical recognition programs to assure that staff were being truthful in their narratives. St. Luke's Hospital and Aurora Health Care specifically required "coaching" and "process review" to verify that the narratives reflected the actual, current practice of the staff. That is, one of the functions of the coach was to provide external validation of the narratives as reflections of actual patient care situations. In addition, the process reviewer, who was a member of the shared governance councilor structure, ensured that the staff member and coach indicated that the narratives reflected the staff member's current practice.

Members of the staff, administration, and human resource departments at all three organizations reported that they had grown in their appreciation of the internal validity of the novice to expert models as they worked through the strategies. They saw the models as credible and believed they accurately reflected the developmental growth continuum of health care professionals in their respective institutions.

EXTERNAL VALIDITY, TRANSFERABILITY, AND FITTINGNESS

Transferability is the equivalent of external validity and is the extent to which the conclusions from one setting might be relevant to other contexts (Lincoln and Guba, 1985). This characteristic is sometimes referred to as the "fit" or usefulness of the findings to contexts beyond the current setting. Thick description is one strategy used to assure the transferability of the findings. Thick description is the illustration of theoretical constructions and relationships with direct quotations from the data.

In each of the novice to expert models, the narrators used characteristics of practice to illustrate the domains, that is, behavioral statements written in terms staff commonly used. Exhibit 3–7, Chapter 3 shows the characteristics of practice for various stages in the caring domain of the CPDM. It is interesting to note that the domains of the models are very similar even though they were independently generated from staff narratives from California, Wisconsin, and Massachusetts (Exhibit 12–1). This replication of findings suggests that the models meet the criteria of transferability and fittingness of content. These domains summarize the "essence of practice" for each discipline, and in combination, for health care.

RELIABILITY, DEPENDABILITY, AND AUDIBILITY

In qualitative research, dependability is concerned with the consistency and repeatability of the data collected from multiple subjects (Kirk and Miller, 1986). Thus, it was critical to ensure that the data were consistent with the experience of clinical staff. The staff developed the narratives at each organization and shared them with the members of their design teams. The teams made notes that identified the emerging characteristics of practice. Next, the teams grouped the characteristics of practice into domains.

For example, Aurora HealthCare's Metro CPDM included the following characteristic of practice: "Collaborates with other caregivers to challenge current practices and synthesizes research findings to develop optimal systems to achieve the most effective patient and family outcomes." This statement was categorized into the collaboration domain as it related to integrating research into practice. The characteristic of practice was derived from the narrative shown in Exhibit 12–2. The teams maintained the records of the processes used to develop the models (that is, creating an audit trail) in each of the participating organizations.

As the models were used in clinical recognition programs, it was important that additional strategies were used to assure that the models were reliably and consistently applied to staff. For example, at St. Luke's Medical Center and Aurora Health Care, three expert staff nurse panel members reviewed a nurse's

Exhibit 12–1 Comparisons of Domains of Practice Between the Novice to Expert Models

Benner's Novice to Expert Model	St. Luke's Medical Center's Clinical Practice Developmental Model	Aurora Health Care's Metro Clinical Practice Developmental Model	Massachusetts General Hospital's Interdisciplinary Professional Practice Model
• Helping role	• Caring	• Caring	• Client-patient relationship
• Teaching-coaching functions		• Patient education and professional development	
• Diagnostic and patient monitoring function	• Clinical knowledge and decision making	• Clinical knowledge and decision making	• Clinical knowledge
• Effective management of rapidly changing situations			
• Administering and monitoring therapeutic interventions and regimens			
• Monitoring and ensuring the quality of health care practices			
• Organizational and work-role competencies	• Collaboration	• Collaboration	• Teamwork and collaboration

Source: Courtesy of Aurora HealthCare-Metro Region, Milwaukee, Wisconsin.

Exhibit 12–2 Narrative Used to Substantiate the Research Characteristic of Practice for the Expert Stage in the Aurora Metro Clinical Practice Developmental Model

"While I was admitting an elderly female to our rehabilitation unit from her home, she relayed to me that she had been having blood-tinged sputum recently. She was not on an anticoagulation medication, and her calves were edematous but non-tender. She was obese and on Premarin and had been very immobile. Her breath sounds were diminished and a pulse ox check read 89 percent on room air. I phoned her primary medical doctor with the information and my suspicion of a pulmonary emboli. He ordered blood gases and they came back abnormal. I phoned her physician again and explained the results. He agreed to a VQ scan which came back with a high probability of a Pulmonary Emboli. She was started on the heparin **protocol (an evidence-based medical practice guideline),** including Zantac 150 mg at bedtime.

I spent a great deal of time explaining the heparin treatment to the patient and her elderly husband. At their request, I then phoned their only daughter and explained the situation to her, as **I knew that education and comprehension were essential to support patient and family coping**.

The next morning, the day after her first day on the heparin drip, it was reported that she had become terribly confused at night, climbed out of bed, and pulled out her IV. She had been started early in the day on the Heparin and showed no problems on my shift or the evening shift. I consulted the pharmacist and was told that neither Zantac or the Ambien she had received at bedtime had the adverse effect of confusion. **I had observed confusion one time before in one of my elderly patients on Zantac, and she had taken the Ambien on the surgical floor and there was no mention in her chart of any confusion**.

I called her physician and explained the night's events and questioned whether Zantac was causing the problem. His reply was that people don't become confused with Zantac, but did give orders for some labs that included a liver panel. Her liver function tests came back very elevated, yet her admission labs were normal.

continues

Exhibit 12–2 continued

I asked the night shift to hold her sleeping pill that night and explained my reasons. That second night, she again became very confused, crawled out of bed, and pulled her IV out a second time. She was very upset the next morning because she had heard staff talk about how confused she was that she needed to have the restraint applied.

I spoke with her and offered some reassurance and told her my suspicion that I felt it was a medication that was causing her to become confused at night. She seemed to be a little relieved with that explanation. I phoned her physician again and relayed the episode of confusion to him again, *only this time, I was able to tell him that we had not given her the sleeping pill and that the only medication she had received at bedtime was the Zantac.* He agreed to stop the Zantac. That night she slept soundly and she was much relieved in the morning to find out she did not climb out of bed again. Her physician was surprised to learn that she had slept well that night. He then ordered another liver panel in two days. The enzyme levels came back almost normal.

Several days later, her physician came up to me and complimented me on "my call with the pulmonary emboli and my persistence with the Zantac." *I thanked him and encouraged him to fill out a form for the pharmacy reporting confusion as a potential adverse effect of Zantac,* which I just happened to have on my clipboard. (I had hoped to talk further with him regarding this and this was a perfect opportunity.) He agreed to fill the form out, but *I also reported my findings to the pharmacist so that she could follow-up and make sure everything was reported. Since this patient, I have noted two other patients who have had varying degrees of confusion with Zantac and was able to spot it much quicker.* My patient completed a rather uneventful rehab stay and was discharged to home with a new drug adverse reaction, Zantac.

—Laurel Wilson, RN, Clinical Practice Nurse Stage 5
2CEF, St. Luke's Medical Center, Milwaukee, WI

The bolded italics indicate areas coded as evidence of research-based practice associated with the characteristic of practice for expert collaboration in the Aurora Health Care Metro Clinical Practice Development Model.

Source: Courtesy of Aurora HealthCare-Metro Region, Milwaukee, Wisconsin.

narratives independently and came to consensus on the nurse's stage of development, from novice to expert. The expert panel interviewed the nurse to clarify issues. Subsequently, on the basis of the additional data the nurse provided, the expert panel made a decision about the nurse's staging. (See Chapter 5 for a more thorough discussion of the staging process.) An additional expert staff nurse from one of the shared governance councils reviewed the decisions of the panel and confirmed that all procedural steps of the promotion process were followed.

Staff could appeal the panels' and council's decision. From June 1993 to December 1997, St. Luke's expert panels have met with 1,220 nurses. Table 9–1 shows the outcome of the staging process. During that four-year period, the appeals rate has been less than 2 percent annually, indicating the high inter-rater reliability of the staging process.

SUMMARY OF VALIDITY AND RELIABILITY ISSUES

Design committees and implementation groups can use these strategies to assure that the models generated from narratives are representative of staff practice and that the models are applied consistently over time. Sharing the derivation of elements and domains within the models with an organization's staff, administration, and human resource personnel usually allays concerns about the validity and reliability of the models and their use.

FUTURE DIRECTIONS FOR RESEARCH

As organizations begin to use novice to expert models, rich descriptions of clinical practice become available for study. Many research questions can be raised and answered by examining the staffs' narrative and interview data. Those who have been involved with implementing novice to expert models have asked a refined set of questions and are designing studies to answer some of these. Research questions include:

- What is the linguistic evidence that distinguishes the unique contribution of each discipline to the achievement of quality patient outcomes?

- What is the linguistic evidence of "best practice" in interdisciplinary models and how do we promote the continued growth of interdisciplinary best practice over time?
- What is the effect on patient outcomes of creating staffing schedules so that every patient has ongoing access to expert care?
- To what extent do our documentation systems reflect the expert care that is delivered?
- What personal and environmental resources strengthen professional developmental growth over time?
- How do novice to expert models evolve as practice evolves?

This last question is the most important for us all. Gordon cautioned potential users of formal models such as the novice to expert model:

> [T]heir reductionism, their elemental approach, their explicitness, their objectivity, are exactly what is desired in some situations. In others, however, they work against the goals and intents of the users, such as indirectly restricting autonomy among staff by legislating action...Let formal models in many cases be regarded as training wheels, essential for the first safe rides, unnecessary and limiting once replaced by greater skill. Let not reality be confused with the model. And let us not forget that the model is a tool, not a mirror (Gordon, 1984).

CONCLUSION

In conclusion, we need to continue to study the essence of clinical practice and seek the answers to the above questions as we continue our efforts to evolve best practices. The essence of health care that has evolved in the last decade consists of clinical knowledge, caring, collaboration, patient education, and professional development. Clinical practice will continue to evolve. Excellence in research can guide this evolution to its ultimate aim: creating expert practitioners to deliver quality patient care.

REFERENCES

Benner, P. (1984). *From novice to expert: Excellence and power in clinical nursing practice.* Menlo Park, CA: Addison-Wesley.

Gordon D.R. (1984). Research applications: Identifying the use and misuse of formal models in nursing practice. In P. Benner (Ed.), *From novice to expert* (pp. 225–243). Menlo Park, CA: Addison-Wesley.

Haag-Heitman, B., & Kramer, A. (1998). Creating a Clinical Practice Developmental Model. *American Journal of Nursing,* 98(8), 39–43.

Kirk, J. & Miller, M.L. (1986). *Reliability and validity in qualitative research.* Beverly Hills, CA: Sage.

Ladewig, N.E., Haag, B.J., & Webber, B.T. (1994). The Clinical Practice Development Model: a framework for the recognition of nursing practice. *Aspen's Advisor for Nurse Executives,* 9(4), 5–7.

Lincoln, Y.S., & Guba, E.G. (1985). *Naturalistic inquiry.* Beverly Hills, CA: Sage.

Miles, M.B., & Huberman, A.M. (1994). *Qualitative data analysis* (2nd ed.). Thousand Oaks, CA: Sage.

Polit, D.F., & Hungler, B.P., (1995). *Nursing Research: Principles and Methods.* Philadelphia: J.B. Lippincott Co.

Nuccio, S.A., Lingen, D., Burke, L.J., et al. (1996). The Clinical Practice Developmental Model: The transition process. *Journal of Nursing Administration,* 26(12), 29–37.

Chapter 13

The Role of the Chief Nurse Executive in Fostering Excellence in the Professional Practice Environment

Vicki George

A NEW CONTEXT FOR ORGANIZATIONS

It is a new age for the leadership of today. Rapid advances in technology, global marketing, and the information age have forced leaders to respond or face the eviction of their companies. The successful business of the future can no longer be built around an infrastructure of hierarchical and bureaucratic decision making. In order for success to occur, the business of today must switch from an organization in which there is a handful of bosses at the top who make all the decisions while mindless workers carry out production orders (Drucker, 1992), to an organization that requires its leaders and workers to share in a common mission for the future.

This shared vision needs to account for changing demographics in the workforce and the movement from a manufacturing to a service-based economy. This shared vision requires leaders and workers to put infrastructures in place that foster freedom-oriented decision making at point of services. The consumer is demanding this freedom of action at point of service and the new knowledge worker is capable of implementing it. The new work of leadership is to coach this responsibility-based decision making. By facilitating its successful implementation, customer loyalty will ensure an organization's long-term financial success (Bell, 1998; Boyett & Boyett, 1995).

The health care business is no different. The same political and economic forces have transformed an industry based on an "illness" to an industry based on "wellness." A movement away from an emphasis on acute care toward an emphasis on integrated delivery systems places increased demand on management to drive decisions to the place where the knowledge worker and the consumer interact. The patients are demanding a voice in the decisions that impact their care and on the outcomes they want for themselves and their family. Consumers are demanding a partnership arrangement where information about care is shared between patient and provider. As the health care system responds to these demands, the role of nursing becomes of paramount importance. Nurse leaders of newly created integrated health systems will require a new level of accountability from the professional staff. Maintaining the knowledge of those who practice and fostering a higher level of autonomy to act upon that clinical knowledge is the new work of nursing. The new work of nursing leadership will be to build decision-making models that foster this professionalism.

THE ROLE OF THE CHIEF NURSE EXECUTIVE

With 1.6 million employed professional nurses in the United States, of whom two thirds work at hospitals, it would appear that the place to begin the change is in the hands of the nurse leaders in hospital settings. The chief nurse executive (CNE) or vice president of nursing has typically been seen as a critical element for success in the process of change. The CNE plays a pivotal role because he or she is both an administrator and a professional nurse. The administrative component of the role is grounded in the principles of management and the nurse role should foster the professional ethics of nursing as a discipline. It is the marriage of these two philosophies that makes the CNE's contribution to health care administration unique.

If the ultimate contribution of the CNE is to facilitate the establishment of a professional practice environment that fosters clinical excellence and expert nursing practice, then the marriage of these two roles is critical to the success of the nursing organization. The CNEs must recognize that in their positions they hold a dual accountability, one to the organization's goals and the second to the ethics of professionalism. The CNE plays a vital role in educating the organization to the needs of the profession and in educating the professional to the goals of the organization. Marrying the needs of the organization into a set of goals that can balance the professional's need for autonomy is the principle that will define a new shared vision.

If we are to understand this marriage or partnership, we must first understand the theoretical underpinning of the professionalism and the framework for leadership that will foster the professional's growth and participation. As with any marriage, finding the common ground or interest upon which to build mutual trust will facilitate the goal of sharing in the decision-making process. The CNE must learn to trust the professional to make autonomous decisions at point of service, and in turn, the professional must learn to trust the CNE to make organizational or system decisions that foster quality patient outcomes.

THE ROLE OF THE PROFESSIONAL NURSE

If nurses are to be recognized as true professionals, they must own the accountabilities inherent in the professionalism of the discipline. The creation of an environment of professional practice requires that the decision makers understand the theoretical underpinnings of professionalism. Building the components of what creates a professional into the professional practice environment promotes the concept of professionalism, which in return builds excellence in clinical practice. This is the fundamental role of nursing and nursing leaders.

The theoretical underpinning for the professionalism of nursing is divided from the sociology of professions and models for accommodating professionals in organizations. The literature on the sociology of professions delineates conditions for the practice of a profession and claims that professional practice can occur within bureaucratic organizations when the necessary conditions are met.

Moore (1970) describes a profession as an occupation whose incumbents create and explicitly use systematically accumulated general knowledge in the solution of problems presented by the clientele (either individuals or collective) (p. 56). Carr-Saunders and Wilson made the first attempt in 1933 to analyze a profession. They asserted that a professional tradition raises the ethical standards and widens the social outlook.

A number of sociologists building on the work of Carr-Saunders and Wilson have identified more defined characteristics of a profession-to-be:

1. A commitment to a calling, which is demonstrated by members of the occupation subscribing to established expectations for the behavior of the persons in the occupation (Greenwood, 1957; Gross, 1958; Moore, 1970).
2. Identification with peers, especially in some formalized professional organization (Greenwood, 1957; Gross, 1958; Moore, 1970).
3. Organization around a body of knowledge (Goode, 1969; Greenwood, 1957; Gross, 1958; Hall, 1969; Moore, 1970).
4. Autonomy to use one's own judgment and authority, restraint by responsibility (Greenwood, 1957; Moore, 1970).

A central characteristic of a profession is the degree of personal involvement with clients, which is included by some as part of the service orientation. The mechanisms for credentialing, selection of staff knowledge development, and peer review of the individual and collective practice underscores the professional's service commitment (Mass, 1977).

THE ROLE OF PROFESSIONALS IN ORGANIZATIONS

An organization can be defined as a collective that is goal-oriented, is open to the environment, has boundaries, technologies, structures and processes, and performs activities in varying degrees of effectiveness and efficiency (Zeyferrell, 1979). Organizations vary in the amount of power or control exercised by one set of participants over another, and also in their total amount of control exercised by the participants (Tannenbaum, 1968). Issues of control and participation are of concern to persons working in organizations, particularly to professionals who seek control of their practice as a professional

(Jacox, 1971). The traditional structure for a complex organization is bureaucracy. In the bureaucratic model, management controls professionals and determines the scope of worker participation in decision making. Policies, procedures and guidelines are provided to the worker as a way to control and avoid variations in procedural outcomes. The bureaucratic model applies very well to organizations in stable environments with well-understood technologies. There appears little need in these types of organizations for professional adaptation and learning (Burns and Stalkner, 1961).

One problem with these bureaucratic organizations is that because the control of resources and evaluation of the profession come through the vertical chain of command and control, the cooperation or team work that occurs horizontally is perceived as less important and therefore impaired by the structure itself (Benvenista, 1987). In hospital structures, professionals tend to have many lateral interdependencies and need to work more in the horizontal communication and cooperation aspects. As professionals develop within organizations, conflict also results between the bureaucratic model and that of the highly developed independent professional (Hughes, 1963). In the traditional bureaucratic organization, there is a high degree of centralization of authority and formalization of roles and procedures. These processes in hospitals can interfere with the individual's professional use of specialized knowledge to solve client problems. There are reasons for the concern around organizational arrangements that impact on professional autonomy. Structures for decision making should be developed to work toward providing autonomy at the point of service. Hall (1969) suggests that the presence of professionals in organizations affects the structure of the organization and at the same time the organization affects the work of the professional. Conflicts that occur typically develop over the professional's desire and need for autonomy to carry out their work, and the managers desire to maintain the organization's directives (i.e. resource control). One could envision an answer to the conflict might be a structural model of decision making where an aggregate of talented professionals shares their professional goals as a way to incorporate them into the organizational goals. If such a structure could evolve, the professional and the organization could develop a common vision whereby the organizational goals and the professional goals are aligned in ways that create a positive outcome for the client and the public. There are many models in the literature that have been developed to accommodate professionals within an organizational structure (Benvenista, 1987, Porter-O'Grady, 1992). It is imperative that the leaders and the followers within the organization come to some common direction in terms of how that structure not only should be developed, but who should do the developing. In addition, there must be a clear understanding going forward about what power and authority rests with the organization and what power and authority is placed in the hands of the professional.

NURSING AS A PROFESSION

Nursing is identified by sociologists as a semi-profession (Etzioni, 1969 and Goode, 1969), as an emerging profession (Merton, 1960), and a profession in process (Wilensky, 1964). Nursing's current status as a semi-profession or an emerging profession is consistent with the fear of the process by which professionalization occurs. Nursing is among one of the newer groups to have grown substantially as a consequence of large-scale, hospital organizational structures. It never enjoyed a free state as a profession. The increased demand for nursing services did not automatically result in nursing's increased development as a profession. Professionalization in nursing is progressing in the area of competence and in the achievement of autonomy for control over the practice of nurses. Nurses need increased authority and power in the health care arena to realize the potential benefits for clients from their service.

As stated earlier, nursing management in organizations, and particularly the CNE, have been developed over the past decades as an early attempt to give nurses as professionals this increased authority and control over the practice of nursing. This model of management was built on the study of leadership that in many ways has only been the study of leaders and the context in which they lead (Bass & Stogdill, 1990). Most theories describe the leader's traits or the situational variables that affect the action of the leader. However, Kelley (1992) suggests that effective followers are critical for a leader's or an organization's success because followers, not leaders, determine at least eighty percent of what gets done in organizations.

This concept holds true for hospitals as organizations. Eighty percent of the work that gets done is ordered by physicians and implemented by nurses. Since physicians do not typically have an employed relationship with hospital administration, it is the nurse as a professional who is most impacted by the leader-follower equation. If nursing management models have been developed in the tradition of hierarchical, bureaucratic decision making, the need for a more decentralized decision making approach to point of service delivery is driving the need for these existing structures to change. A new model of leadership must emerge: shared leadership or shared governance.

The degree of professional autonomy granted as an occupational group is dependent upon the success of its efforts to establish a self-governance network (Aydelotte, 1983). The establishment of governance structures that increase nurse autonomy and accountability within organizations is one method to assure this goal.

Since nurses are at the core of this health care system strategic resource (AONE, 1992), nurses will need to demonstrate increased levels of knowledge in their practice and of their practice. In turn, nurses need to feel an increased level of support for the freedom to take the action necessary to affect positive outcomes for the clients they serve.

NURSING SHARED GOVERNANCE

Governance, which has been defined as establishment and maintenance of social, political, and economic arrangements by which practitioners maintain control over their practice, self-discipline, working conditions, and professional affairs, is an antecedent to autonomy (Mass & Specht, 1994). Autonomy is the attribute that is needed to affect professional practice within an organization (Aydelotte, 1983). Nursing shared governance is a model of partnership versus hierarchy in which nurses, employees and the organization form a partnership to meet the goals of the organization and the mandates of the nursing profession (Porter-O'Grady, 1991). Nursing shared governance creates an environment of equals in which nurses at every level of the organization play a role in the decisions that affect nursing activity throughout the organization. Governance or control is at the core of the system and authority and accountability are shared by all registered nursing staff (Porter-O'Grady, 1991). Implementation of nurse shared governance is a developmental process that gives the nurse collective in the organization. It requires the development of new processes and structures, and new roles for nursing staff and management, that will contribute to an environment that supports autonomy and accountability for individual and collective practice. Coupled with the need for this evolution of development in which nursing shared governance is implemented, is the need for the identification of decision-making authority around such parameters as nursing practice. The mechanisms for joint management and staff nurse decision making become the development of models such as shared decision making or shared leadership. Participation in decision making, empowerment, and professional practice are the principles that must be developed and maintained if models of shared governance are to be successful.

PEER REVIEW AND PROFESSIONAL PRACTICE

Autonomy is the ultimate attribute required for the identification of a professional. The degree to which the professional is personally involved with the decisions that impact at point of service is also the degree to which society or the organization places trust in them as a profession.

Although educational and licensing requirements are meant to ensure this trust with society, these mechanisms by virtue of their process can only ensure minimum competencies of the professional. For a professional in an organized setting, the work of membership is to provide ongoing control of the work of its members to ensure an outcome that is in the best interest of their clients. As specialization increases, so must the relative autonomy of the professional to judge the measurement of its practice. Outsiders cannot judge the expert content knowledge of the professional. The most effective control of professional knowledge and level of professional practice is from a peer group of colleagues.

Peer review in organizations is not an easy task. Their review is sometimes complicated by loyalty among professionals to one another. Peer review can be complicated by the need to protect the privacy of the client while examining the client's care. Peer review can be difficult in that essential behaviors must be able to be recognized, even if not observable by peers.

Regardless of these complicating factors, a peer review system must be developed if a professional is to maintain control of his or her practice. Some system of peer evaluation must be developed to demonstrate to the organization and to the public that, as professionals, they hold themselves accountable for the services they provide. The process cannot be confused with a managerial goal review process, but it must coexist with the organization's evaluation process.

If the CNE is to be successful in facilitating the development of a professional practice environment, some model of shared leadership incorporating peer review must exist. The model must assure the ongoing monitoring of the care provided at point of service, and the care provider delivering the service. Through this model the accountability for peer review must rest in the hands of the professionals engaged in the work. It must be a model of peer review that is supported with both financial and human resources. It must be a model that aligns the parameters of care delivered by the provider with the service goals developed by the organization.

Such a peer review model was created at St. Luke's Medical Center. The nurses and nursing leadership at St. Luke's Medical Center took on the challenge of creating a shared vision. The vision was based on a common understanding of what it means to be a professional and what it takes to create a professional's practice environment. The staff nurses, through an account-ability-based decision-making model of shared governance, took on the goal of creating a peer review process that was built on clinical excellence in practice. They chose narratives as a way to describe and measure the care and the care provider. Reading narratives and defining the characteristics of practice provided the framework for the Clinical Practice Development Model (CPDM).

BUILDING FOR EXCELLENCE IN PATIENT CARE

As a leader, it is important to recognize that the interrelation-ship of management and staff needs changing. The key to unlocking the leadership question of "What does it take to cre-ate excellence in a professional's practice environment?" rests in the knowledge that the relationship between autonomy and interdependence between the worker and the workplace is for-ever altered.

Identifying the following unfolding realities that are altering the circumstances of how we work is also important:

- Knowledge is a powerful force and the key tool of produc-tion in our service economy (Porter-O'Grady, 1991).
- Clinical knowledge does not rest with the hierarchical lead-ership any more, but is owned by the professional, who is the key to expert service delivery.
- The key predictor of success is how leadership manages this relationship.

For the CNE, the management of this relationship rests in the knowledge that leading a professional staff means letting go of authority for clinical decisions. It means developing a model of decision making that fosters accountability and autonomy by the professional. It means building a foundation of trust from which all else will follow.

REFERENCES

American Organization of Nurse Executives. (1992). The role and functions of the hospital nurse manager. American Organization of Nurse Executives. *Nursing Management*, 23(9),36–8.

Aydelotte, M.K. (1983). Professional nursing: the driver for governance. In N.L. Chaska (Ed.), *The nursing profession: a time to speak* (pp. 830–843). New York: McGraw-Hill.

Bass, B.M. & Stogdill, R.M. (1990). *Bass and Stogdill's handbook on leadership: theory, research and managerial applications* (3rd ed.). New York: Free Press

Bell, C. (1998). *Managing customer loyalty.* Presentation to Aurora HealthCare Board, Milwaukee, WI.

Benvenista, G. (1987). *Professionalizing the organization: reducing bureaucracy to enhance effectiveness.* San Francisco: Jossey-Bass.

Boyett, J.H. & Boyett, J.T. (1995) *Beyond workplace 2000: essential strategies for the new American corporation.* New York: E.P. Dutton.

Burns, T. & Stalkner, G.M. (1961) *The management of innovation.* London: Tavistock.

Carr-Saunders, A.M., & Wilson, P.A. (1933). *The professions.* Oxford, England: Clarendon Press.

Drucker, P. (1992) The new society of organization. *Harvard Business Review*, 70(5), 95–104.

Etzioni, A. (1969). *Semi-professions and their organizations.* New York: Free press.

Greenwood. (1957). Attributes of a profession. *Social Work*, 2(3), 44–45.

Goode, W.J. (1969). The theoretical limits of professionalization. In A. Etsion, (Ed.), *The semi-professions and their organization: teaching nurses and social workers.* New York: The Free Press, pp. 266–313.

Gross, E. (1958). *Work and society.* New York: Thomas & Cromwell.

Hall, R.H. (1969). *Occupations and the social structure.* Englewood Cliffs, NJ: Prentice-Hall.

Hughes, E. (1963). Professions. *Daedalus*, 92(3),655–688

Jacox, A. (1971). Collective action in control of practice by professionals. *Nursing Forum*, 10(3),239–257.

Kelley, R.E. (1992). *The power of followership: how to create leaders people want to follow and followers who lead themselves.* New York: Currency/ Doubleday.

Mass, M.L. (1977). *Guidelines for nurse autonomy/patient welfare.* New York: Appleton-Century-Crofts.

Mass, M.L., & Specht, J. (1994). Shared governancy in nursing: what is shared? who governs? and who benefits? In J. McCloskey & H. Grace (Eds.). *Current Issues in Nursing* (4th ed.).(pp. 398–409). St. Louis: Mosby.

Merton, R.K. (1960). The search for professional status. *American Journal of Nursing*, 60(5), 662.

Moore, W.E. (1970). *The professions: roles and rules.* New York: Russell Sage Foundation.

Porter-O'Grady, T. (1991). Shared governance for nursing; part I: creating the new organization. *AORN Journal*, 53(2), 458–466.

Porter-O'Grady, T., (1992). *Implementing shared governance, creating a professional organization.* St. Louis: Mosby.

Tannenbaum, a.S. (1968). *Control in organization.* New York: McGraw-Hill.

Wilensky, H.L. (1964). The professional and everyone. *American Journal of Sociology*, 79, 137–158.

Zeyferrell, M. (1979). *Dimensions of organizations.* Santa Monica, CA: Goodyear Publishing Co.

From Career Ladder
to
Clinical Practice Development
Model (CPDM):
A Timeline at a Glance

Clinical Practice Development Model at a Glance

1989

JUNE, 1989
Peer Review Committee of PNA began looking at career ladder.

SEPTEMBER, 1989
Consultations with Tim Porter O'Grady and shared governance task force.

1990

JANUARY, 1990
Peer Review Committee sets goal to evaluate various career ladder models from other institutions.

JUNE, 1990
Peer Review Committee began review of six career ladders from other institutions.

OCTOBER, 1990
Last meeting of PNA Committees.

DECEMBER, 1990
Reorganization of shared governance to a councilar model. Election of housewide councils.

1991

JANUARY, 1991
Initiation of housewide councilar model.

MAY, 1991
Councils define specific accountibilities.

AUGUST, 1991
Practice Council completed Nursing Philosophy and Conceptual Framework. Contains Benner's work of novice to expert.

NOVEMBER, 1991
Initial consultation with Benner Associates.

continues

1992   *Benner Associates Consult with PNA Councils Throughout the Year.*

JANUARY, 1992	FEBRUARY, 1992	JUNE, 1992	NOVEMBER, 1992	DECEMBER, 1992
Nursing Practice Council initiates Benner Consult.	Narrative Workgroup starts reading narratives submitted by St. Luke's staff nurses in order to define common themes and characteristics of practice.	Practice Council defines criteria for annual performance review.	Nursing Quality Assessment Council defines process for annual performance review.	Nursing Quallity Assessment Council implements process for annual performance review.
Steering Committee formed to coordinate council and activities for new peer review process.				
Practice Council calls for RN representative from each unit.				
Practice Council calls up Narrative Workgroup.				

continues

1993
July, 1993
Implementation Workgroup completes policy for CPDM transition.

1994
May, 1994
Transition period for CPDM completed with over 700 staged.

July, 1993
First CPDM panels.

August, 1993
Confirmation of staging for the first 11 nurses by the Quality Council.

September, 1993
Nursing Research begins development of research proposal related to CPDM.

Transition period for staging continues until May 1994.

Professional Nursing Assembly Diagram and Bylaws

PROFESSIONAL NURSING ASSEMBLY DIAGRAM

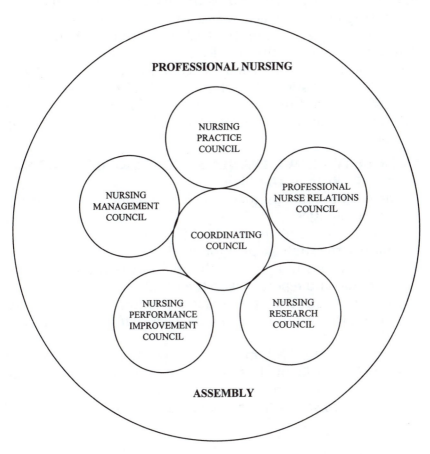

Source: Courtesy of St. Luke's Medical Center, Milwaukee, Wisconsin.

Excerpts from PNA BYLAWS

ARTICLE I—PREAMBLE

The Division of Nursing supports the following articles which provide a framework for the shared governance structure in which practice accountability and autonomy take place at the professional staff nurse level. The shared governance structure is known as The Professional Nurse Assembly, hereafter referred to in these bylaws as the "PNA." The PNA supports the accountability-based practice of nursing to serve both patients and society at large. The PNA is the decision making structure for nursing practice issues in the units/departments identified in the nursing plan of care. The PNA has the authority to create, change or restructure the practice of nursing and the standards of care for the patients. The practice of nursing will be consistent with the mission of St. Luke's Medical Center, the mandates of the Board of Directors, the conceptual framework for nursing practice, and the directives of regulatory/governing agencies.

ARTICLE IV—GOVERNANCE STRUCTURE OF THE PNA
Section 1. Role of the PNA
A. Direct the councils to define and communicate nursing accountabilities.
B. Review, revise and approve PNA bylaws.
C. Approve the strategic plan for nursing.
D. Identify issues and direct to the appropriate council for consideration and report back to the PNA.
E. Provide the structure for interaction among nursing personnel and with administration, medical staff or other individuals.
F. Elect, by vote, PNA members to positions on housewide councils, President-elect and Nominating Committee. (See article regarding process)
G. The council year will run from January to January.

Source: Courtesy of St. Luke's Medical Center, Milwaukee, Wisconsin.

Section 2. Design

A. *Governing Councils*

The PNA conducts the work of developing house wide patient care programs and policies that describe the use of the nursing process executive through five governing councils. These five councils are housewide and known as the governing councils. They are: Nursing Practice Council, Nursing Performance Improvement Council (formerly known as the Nursing Quality Assessment Council), Nursing Research Council, Professional Nurse Relations Council and Nursing Management Council. These five councils are linked together via the Nursing Coordinating Council.

B. *Functional Councils*

All Nursing areas listed in the Plan of Care will design unit based models consistent with the framework of the housewide governing councils. These unit based councils are known as the functional councils. The nursing areas will define the mechanism used to address the accountabilities of the Nursing Practice Council, Nursing Performance Improvement Council, Professional Nurse Relations Council and Nursing Research Council at the unit level. The design of nursing unit councils will be consistent with PNA principles, will reflect nursing staff resources and will include a communication pathway to appropriate governing councils as needed by the units.

Section 3. Council Authority and Accountability

The five governing councils are designed to direct the overall nursing care through mechanisms that allow for unit specific approaches to patient care within the conceptual framework for nursing practice.

A. Nursing Practice Council (NPC)

1. *Definition:*
   The Nursing Practice Council defines the practice of nursing at St. Luke's Medical Center. The Nursing Practice Council has the authority and accountability for establishing and maintaining the standards of practice

and the policies and procedures which describe and guide the nursing care provided. The Council sets the criteria for characteristics of practice required of nurses caring for patients at St. Luke's Medical Center.

2. *Accountabilities:*
   — Operationalizes the conceptual framework for nursing practice.
   — Approves the clinical standards of nursing practice.
   — Defines roles based on accountabilities of nursing care providers.

3. *Membership:*
   Elected Membership to this council concists of: eight (8) Staff Nurses, one (1) Clinical Nurse Specialist/Nurse Clinician and one (1) Nursing Management Representative.

4. *Meetings:*
   The Nursing Practice Council meets a minimum of quarterly.

B. Nursing Performance Improvement Council: (NPIC)
(formerly the Nursing Quality Assessment Council)

1. *Definition:*
   The NPIC has the authority and accountability for evaluating and measuring the quality of the nursing care delivered and for evaluating and measuring the quality of the nursing care provider. This council develops the Nursing Quality Plan of Care that identifies the mechanisms and processes to monitor, evaluate and improve nursing care delivery. This council develops the mechanisms and processes that evaluate nursing care givers performance, competence and growth.

2. *Accountabilities:*
   — Measures the quality of nursing care delivered by providers based on their roles and accountabilities as defined by the Nursing Practice Council.
   — Measures the quality of professional nursing care provided by Registered Nurses via performance review

and via evaluation of growth and development along the clinical practice development model.
— Measures the quality of nursing care delivered through current care delivery systems and evaluates for improvement.

3. *Membership:*
Elected membership to this council consists of: five (5) Staff Nurses, one (1) Clinical Nurse Specialist/Nurse Clinician, and one (1) Nursing Management Representative. The Nursing Support Supervisor is a standing member of this council.

4. *Meetings:*
The Nursing Performance Improvement Council meets a minimum of quarterly.

C. **Nursing Research Council (NRC)**

1. *Definition:*
The Nursing Research Council has the authority and accountability for validation of current nursing practice as well as development of new knowledge related to the nursing care provided or the nursing care providers. This council establishes the professional atmosphere in which nurses are expected to perform using research based practice and promote nursing research activities through definitive educational offerings, communications and resources.

2. *Accountabilities:*
— Validate current nursing knowledge.
— Generate new knowledge and make recommendations for change.
— Assure the ethical conduct of nursing research.

3. *Membership:*
Elected membership to this council consists of: five (5) Staff Nurses, one (1) Clinical Nurse Specialist/Nurse Clinician and one (1) Nursing Management Representative. The occupant of the Walter Schroeder St. Luke's Chair for

Nursing Research and the Director of Nursing Research are standing members of this council.

4. *Meetings:*

The Nursing Research Council meets a minimum of quarterly.

D. Professional Nurse Relations Council (PNRC)

1. *Definition:*

The Professional Nurse Relations Council has the authority and accountability for the education of and communication among the nursing staff members of the Professional Nursing Assembly. This council coordinates nursing recognition events and assists staff members to develop in their nursing practice both within and beyond the organization based on the conceptual framework for education.

2. *Accountabilities:*

— **Professional Relations:** promotes professional nurse image, promotes retention of nursing staff and collaboration with other health care disciplines.
— **Education:** Maintains an educational framework for education programs.
— **Communication:** Operationalizes, maintains and evaluates communication systems for shared governance.
— **Consultation Services:** Coordinates the scope of services provided by SLMC Nursing Consultation Services.

3. *Membership:*

Elected membership to this council counsists of: four (4) Staff Nurses, two (2) Clinical Nurse Specialist/Nurse Clinicians and two (2) Nursing Management Representatives. The Aurora Director of Education is a standing member of this council.

4. *Meetings:*

The Professional Nurse Relations Council meets a minimum of quarterly.

E. The Nursing Management Council (NMC)

1. Definition:

The Nursing Management Council has the authority and accountability to provide for the management of resources as defined in the conceptual framework for nursing management. This council examines the delivery of patient care as it is affected by the availability of human, fiscal, materials, support and systems linkage resources. This council promotes the responsible and creative use of resources so that expenses are controlled while exceeding the health care expectations of the patients and their significant others.

2. *Accountabilities:*
   — **Human Resources:** Operationalizes optimal patient care delivery teams.
   — **Fiscal:** Balances quality care with fiscal responsibility.
   — **Materials Management:** Maximizes resource utilization.
   — **Support:** Creates and maintains an environment consistent with the nursing management philosophy and conceptual framework.
   — **System Linkage:** Collaborate with other departments and disciplines to maximize cost effective, quality patient care.

3. *Membership:*
   Elected membership to this council consists of: six (6) elected members from the Nursing Management Representatives, the Director of Nursing Operations, the PNA President, and one (1) elected member from the Clinical Nurse Specialist/Nurse Clinician group.

4. *Meetings:*
The Nursing Management Council meets a minimum of quarterly.

F. Nursing Coordinating Council (NCC)

1. *Definition:*
The Nursing Coordinating Council provides direction and advice to the five governing councils as needed. It serves to link the five councils together and is the vehicle for the Chief Nursing Executive to participate in activities required to assure hospital wide actions related to the provision of nursing care.

2. *Accountabilities:*
   — Define the goals for the nursing division of St. Luke's Medical Center.
   — Review and prepare the PNA bylaws for presentation to the membership annually.

3. *Membership:*
Elected Membership to this council consists of: the chairs of the five governing councils, the President and President-Elect of the PNA. The Director of Nursing Operations and the Chief Nursing Executive of St. Luke's Medical Center are standing members of this council.

4. *Meetings:*
The Nursing Coordinating Council will meet a minimum of quarterly.

Appendix C

Clinical Practice Development Model

Clinical Practice Development Model
Stage 1

DEFINITION

The Stage 1 novice nurse is a new graduate of a RN program and is on orientation. This nurse is obtaining knowledge and experience in clinical and technical skills. Under the guidance of a preceptor, the nurse collects objective data according to guidelines and rules obtained from nursing education and in orientation. The novice nurse utilizes this objective data and seeks assistance in making clinical decisions.

CARING

1. Responds to comfort needs of patients and families.
2. Recognizes their own feelings in patient/family relationships.

CLINICAL KNOWLEDGE AND DECISION MAKING

1. Learning the hospital's policies, procedures and standards which guide their clinical practice.
2. Needs assistance with correlating theoretical knowledge to clinical situations.
3. Obtaining knowledge and experience in technical skills and needs assistance when performing new skills.
4. Needs assistance in determining priorities of tasks to be completed.

COLLABORATION

1. Practices with the guidance of the preceptor.
2. Beginning to cope with the reality of their own practice.
3. Developing first professional relationships within the health care team.

Source: Courtesy of St. Luke's Medical Center, Milwaukee, Wisconsin.

Clinical Practice Development Model
Stage 2

DEFINITION

Stage 2 advanced beginners are guided by pollicies, procedures and standards. They are building a knowledge base through practice and are most comfortable in a task environment. They describe a clinical situation from the viewpoint of what they need to do, rather than relating the context of the situation or how the patient responds. Advanced beginners practice from a theoretical knowledge base while they recognize and provide for routine patient needs.

CARING

1. Approach patients and families with compassion.
2. Provide comfort for patients.
3. Recognize the importance of therapeutic relationships.
4. Are discovering the appropriate boundaries of therapeutic relationships.

CLINICAL KNOWLEDGE AND DECISION MAKING

1. Are beginning to coorelate theoretical knowledge with clinical information.
2. Recognize the importance of knowing about and managing clinical problems.
3. Are beginning to perceive recurrent, meaningful aspects of cllinical situations.
4. Provide care structured by other members of the health care team.

COLLABORATION

1. Seek assistance and support in unfamiliar clinical situations.
2. Validate practice through external sources.
3. Are beginning to identify their contribution as members of the health care team.

Clinical Practice Development Model
Stage 3

DEFINITION

Stage 3 competent nurses integrate theoretical knowledge with cllinical experience in the care of patients and families. Care is delivered utilizing a deliberate, systematic approach and practice is guided by increasing awareness of patterns of patient responses in recurrent situations. These nurses demonstrate mastery of most technical skills, and begin to view clinical situations from a patient and family focus.

CARING
1. Individualize care and begin to recognize personhood of patient and family.
2. Are learning to establish and practice within the boundaries of therapeutic relationships.

CLINICAL KNOWLEDGE AND DECISION MAKING
1. Demonstrate confidence in delivering Standards of Care.
2. Provide care based on conscious, deliberate planning.
3. Understand the expected progression of clinical events based on concrete past experience.
4. Desire to limit the unexpected by managing the environment.
5. Assume an increasing responsibility to advocate for patients and families.

COLLABORATION
1. Recognize their role and function as a member of the health care team.
2. Delegate to other care given as a means to help manage the clinical situation.

Clinical Practice Development Model
Stage 4 Nurses

DEFINITION

Stage 4 nurses are proficient practitioners who have in-depth knowledge of nursing practice, perceived situations as a whole and comprehend the significant elements based on previoius experience. These nurses demonstrate the ability to recognize situational changes that require unplanned or unanticipated interventions. They respond to most situations with confidence, speed and flexibility. Progression is from a tasks orientation to a holistic view of patient care. The nurses develop effective relationships with other caregivers and provide leadership within the health care team to formulate integrated approaches to care. They interpret the patient and family experiences from a perspective that begins to envision and create possibilities.

CARING

1. Establish trsuting therapeutic relationships through understanding of specific and relevant aspects of the patient and family's experiences.
2. Realize the significant impact that life events and health status changes have on patients and families and are able to offer guidance and support.
3. Assist patients and families to identify the implications and possible outcomes of healthcare decisions.
4. Relate to patients and families in a non-judgmental manner and respect their choices.
5. Recognize that healing requires more than physical interventions. They promote an environment grounded in empathy, kindness and a deep regard for the individual. Patient and family strengths are identified and possibilities are recognized.
6. Understand that physical, psychological, social and spiritual needs are interdependent and unique to the patient and family.

7. Utilize increasing levels of family involvement and participation in goal setting, planning, and providing care.
8. Explore creative approaches to advocate for patients and families.

CLINICAL KNOWLEDGE AND DECISION MAKING
1. Perceive the important aspects of a clinical situation and quickly focus in on the accurate region of the problem.
2. Identify situational changes that require actions other than those planned or anticipated.
3. Communicate clearly and delegate effectively in rapidly changing situations.
4. Demonstrate confident use of technology and correlate clinical information to the situation.

COLLABORATION
1. Struggle with ethical/moral dilemmas in relation to own personal feelings.
2. Develop effective relationships with other caregivers and provide leadership within the healthcare team.
3. Mobilize other health care team members to achieve best possible patient outcomes.
4. Assume accountability beyond their direct responsibilities.
5. Recognize conflict and involve themselves to pursue the best patient outcomes.

Clinical Practice Development Model
Stage 5 Nurses

DEFINITION
Stage 5 nurses are an expert practitioner whose intuition and skill arise from comprehensive knowledge grounded in experience. Their practice is characterized by a flexible, innovative and confident self-directed approach to patient and family care. Expert nurses operate from a deep understanding of the total situation. They put into perspective their own personal values and are able to encourage and support patient and family choices. Expert nurses collaborate with other caregivers to challenge and coordinate institutional resources to maximize advocacy for patient and family care in achieving the most effective outcomes.

CARING
1. Presencing: Being with the patient
   a. Establish trusting relationship with patients grounded in a philosophy of "being with" rather than "doing to" a patient. "Being with" is characterized by a mental and emotional presence that evolves from deep feelings for the patient's experience.
   b. Actively listen in an effort to understand, though not necessarily agree with, patient and family choices.
   c. Demonstrate a deep understanding of the unique meaning of health, illness & disease on a patient & family.
2. Giving Hope and Create a Healing Environment
   a. Promote healing by helping the patient & family cope with the fears & concerns that accompany life changes.
   b. Facilitate patient/family decision-making by assuring that adequate information is available.
   c. Assist patient and family in the examination and clarification of their values within the context of the clinical situation.

d. Utilize creative approaches to empower patients and families involving them in goal-setting, planning and providing care.

CLINICAL KNOWLEDGE AND DECISION MAKING
1. Clinical Intuition/Forethought
   a. Possess an intuitive grasp of the clinical situation by recognizing patterns and similarities in a problem without wasteful consideration of a large range of unfruitful possibilities.
   b. Demonstrate exquisite foresight in anticipating problems and intervene before explicit diagnostic signs are evident.
2. Effective Management of Rapidly Changing Situations
   a. Act decisively and delegate effectively in potentially life-threatening situations.
   b. Communicate clearly and convincingly to make the clinical case in order to obtain timely and appropriate responses from physicians.
   c. Maximize patient outcomes in situations which allow only short term or indirect patient contact.
   d. Prioritize quickly in unpredictable situations and adjust strategies accordingly.
3. Diagnostic Monitoring and Decision Making
   a. Selectively apply technology and correlate it to the patient's response.
   b. Critically evaluate own decision-making and judgements.

COLLABORATION
1. Personal Knowledge of Self
   a. Recognize knowledge of self to maintain objectivity and separate personal feelings within ethical/moral situations.
2. Therapeutic Team
   a. Value the expertise of the team members and creatively coordinate resources to provide the highest quality care for patient/family.

      b. Influence practice by challenging the system & expanding boundaries to best meet the patient/family needs.

      c. Identify the dilemma and offer constructive coping strategies.

      d. Negotiate conflict by focusing on patient outcomes and promoting collaboration.

3. Peer Support/Credibility

      a. Provide emotional and situational support for colleagues.

      b. Promote unit stability and encourage teamwork.

      c. Are sought out by colleagues for formal and informal consultation.

      d. Portray a professional image and positively influence practice.

Appendix D

Staging/Advancement Policy for the Clinical Practice Development Model

I. CLINICAL PRACTICE DEVELOPMENT MODEL

The St. Luke's Medical Center Clinical Practice Development Model (CPDM) is based on the novice to expert theory that describes a registered nurse in clinical practice. The RN moves through stages of development from novice to expert based on experience, acquisition of knowledge, and development of skills. Narratives are the means to identify, recognize, and acknowledge nursing practice to determine the stage of development along the growth continuum.

A. Each stage of development contains three domains of practice:
1. Caring
2. Clinical knowledge and decision making
3. Collaboration
Each of these three domains must be represented in the group of three narratives and must support the stage of practice recommended by the CPDM panel.

Source: Courtesy of St. Luke's Medical Center, Milwaukee, Wisconsin.

B. CPDM utilizes a peer review process referred to as the CPDM panel review.

II. STAGING TIMEFRAMES

A. Initial staging of staff RNs is a requirement at SLMC to ensure the quality of the caregiver. NPIC requires these RNs to meet at least stage 2 characteristics in order to practice after orientation and/or take call without an assigned resource person on site. Although all RNs must apply for staging within four to six months of their start date, NPIC recognizes that experienced RNs hired into a distinctly different clinical area may need six to twelve months to realize their full staging potential. NPIC encourages ongoing coaching and application for advancement after initial staging.

B. Initial Staging

1. New Graduate—will submit three clinical narratives within two months of completion of formal orientation or within four months of start date (whichever comes later). They will be held accountable for stage 1 characteristics of practice until NPIC confirmation. New graduates will function with a preceptor or an assigned resource until the staging process is complete and they have achieved at least a stage 2 designation.

2. New Hires with Experience—will submit three clinical narratives within two months of completion of formal orientation or within four months of start date (whichever comes later). New hires with less than one year of clinical experience will be held accountable for stage 1 characteristics of practice until NPIC confirmation. New hires with more than one year of clinical experience will be held accountable for characteristics of stage 2 until NPIC confirmation.

3. Transfers from non-staff RN positions who have not been previously staged must meet the same criteria as the new hire with experience.

C. Advancement

Staff RNs can apply for advancement when all the following criteria are met:

1. Self-assessment reveals individual growth along the continuum into the next stage of development.
2. Annual Performance Review (APR) standards related to professional practice have been met. Refer to the Clinical Nursing Practice Evaluation.
3. There is a professional development plan and/or personal mastery goal(s) in place addressing growth areas identified in any other APR standards. Progress is being demonstrated toward meeting those standards as negotiated between staff RN and manager, CNS/NC.
4. Applicant is not under any disciplinary action.
5. A minimum of six months has passed since the last NPIC confirmation.

III. NARRATIVES

A. Narratives

Narratives define nursing practice by capturing the complexity of the interpersonal, ethical, and clinical judgements of actual nursing practice. Narratives must be reflective of the individual's current practice; therefore, clinical experiences used in the narratives must have occurred in the past year and at least one must be from the current unit of practice at SLMC. All three domains: caring, clinical knowledge and decision making, and collaboration must be evident in the group of three narratives.

B. Falsification

Falsification of clinical narratives will result in disciplinary action as directed by the Nurse Management Council.

C. Portfolio

Each RN applying for staging/advancement will have a portfolio. The portfolio will include:

1. The application form for CPDM Staging/Advancement including the signatures of the coach and the manager.
2. Three clinical narratives reflecting nursing practice occurring in past year and at least one narrative from current unit of practice at SLMC.
3. Narratives submitted must meet the following criteria:
    a. typed standard size and print
    b. double spaced on 8 1/2 × 11 inch paper, one side only, and one inch margins
    c. length may vary but a maximum of five pages per narrative is preferred
    d. employee ID number on all three narratives. No applicant name on or within the narratives
    e. name on application form only
    f. number narrative 1, 2, 3 in upper right hand corner of each narrative.

D. Copies of narratives may be forwarded to other councils if issues are brought forth re: practice/system issues and/or provide valuable information which would contribute toward enhanced understanding of CPDM characteristics.

IV. MANAGER

A. The manager plays an integral role in the CPDM process. The manager may participate in the CPDM process as a coach or as a resource for the applicant and the coach.
B. The manager will be accountable for evaluating the advancement criteria for each applicant (refer to Section II C of this policy).
C. The manager's signature on the application form means that the staging advancement criteria is met (refer to Section II C of this policy). Coaching for the staging/advancement should not begin until the manager signs the application form.

V. COACHING

A. Coaching is a purposeful process. Ideally coaching is the development of an ongoing relationship that provides support and strategies for continued growth in the clinical practice area. Coaching is the role accountability of managers and CNS/NCs. Stage 5 staff nurses may contract with their manager and CNS/NC to participate in coaching specifically for staging as a mechanism to continue their own growth as well as assist others in their growth along the continuum. Coaching for staging is limited to narratives and interview preparation. As an individual determines their readiness for advancement along the CPDM continuum a coach must be utilized.

   B. Coaches Qualifications and Expectations (See Attachment I).

   C. The coach's signature on the application form verifies that:

      1. 1:1 coaching session(s) occurred.

      2. To the best of the coach's knowledge, the clinical situations described, reflect the current clinical practice of the applicant.

VI. APPLICANT ACCOUNTABILITY

   A. Advancement along the CPDM continuum is the accountability of each individual RN.

   B. Eligibility for CPDM staging and advancement requires the following:

      1. The applicant will meet with their manager to discuss advancement/staging plans and to determine whether applicant meets advancement criteria re: Annual Performance Review. (Refer to Section II C of this policy). The manager's signature on the application form is obtained at this time.

      2. The applicant will submit their portfolio to the coach.

      3. The coach and applicant will individually read the narratives and identify the characteristics of practice.

      4. The coach and applicant will have 1:1 session(s) in which they discuss:

         a. the characteristics identified in the narratives and how they relate to the CPDM framework

         b. the interview process and prepare for the interview

5. Ultimately, it is the sole accountability of the applicant to declare one specific stage for which he/she applies.
6. The applicant's signature on the application form verifies that all the processes re: coaching and narratives (refer to Section III of this policy) are in place and adhered to. Failure to comply with these processes may result in return of the applicant's portfolio and possible delay in the staging process.

VII. CPDM PANEL
   A. Scheduling
      1. Panels will be scheduled within the first 2 weeks of each month for the main campus and the third week of the month for St. Luke's South Shore.
      2. Applicants will be scheduled in order of receipt and panel date availability.
      3. The applicant's identity and unit are blinded to the two panel members but not to the facilitator. The panel members will be informed of the stage applied for by the applicant.
      4. The applicant, coach, and PCM will be notified of the CPDM panel date and interview time by the PNA office.
      5. Every attempt will be made to have the applicant staged within two months of application receipt.
      6. Cancellation
         a. cancellations within 10 days of the date indicated on the applicant notification letter, will be rescheduled
         b. cancellation less than 10 days from actual panel date will proceed as scheduled:
            1) if the panel comes to consensus without need for an interview, the staging recommendation will proceed to NPIC for confirmation
            2) if the panel requires an interview to reach a recommendation for staging, then an inter-

view will be scheduled. The applicant attends on their own time

3) the manager will be notified of the late cancellation

B. Panel Composition

1. Each CPDM panel will consist of three staff nurse members selected from a housewide panel pool. One member is the panel facilitator.
2. The three staff nurses (staged at 4 or 5) have been validated in their ability to read narratives and identify characteristics of nursing practice based on the CPDM framework.
3. If application is for stage 4 or 5, at least two panel members will be staff nurses who are stage 5. If application is for stage 2 or 3, the panel makeup may be entirely stage 4 members.
4. A silent 4th member may be present for educational purposes if applicant agreement is obtained prior to convening the panel.

C. Housewide Panel Member Qualifications and Role Expectations (See Attachment II)

D. Housewide Facilitator Qualifications and Role Expectations (See Attachment III)

E. CPDM Facilitator and Panel Member Rotation Policy (See attachment IV)

F. CPDM Panel

1. Each panel member will individually review and stage the three clinical narratives prior to the panel.
2. Panel members will meet at CPDM panel time to discuss the narratives and reach consensus about the characteristics of nursing practice identified. Strategies for interview will be developed to engage the applicant in discussion of their clinical practice.
3. After interview the panel members will strive for consensus for staging recommendations.

4. The recommendation of the panel will be discussed with the applicant and forwarded to NPIC.

5. If the panel's recommendation differs from the applied for stage, options regarding appeal and coach follow-up will be discussed with the applicant.

G. CPDM Interview Process

1. The applicant is greeted and introductions are made identifying the facilitator and the specialty representative, if requested.

2. A brief explanation of the panel's process is reviewed.

3. All three domains and all three narratives are addressed during the course of the interview.

4. The interview is applicant focused and respectful.

5. The interview lasts approximately 30 minutes.

6. Recommendations for a stage include information gained from panel review as well as an interview therefore, applicants are informed of consensus decisions after the interview is completed.

7. Applicant is asked to leave room after interview. Panel members reach consensus regarding a recommended stage and upon return, applicant is informed.

VIII. NPIC ACCOUNTABILITIES

A. Approve CPDM staging/advancement policy decisions.

B. Apply CPDM policy to interpret the action needed in individual circumstances brought before NPIC.

C. Monitor CPDM progress, trends, and direct corrective actions (which include referrals) as needed, either to individuals, units, or councils.

D. Address potential quality of care/system concerns which may be revealed through the panel process.

E. Confirm CPDM staging recommendations.

F. In the event of an appeal, the recommendation of the second panel is submitted to NPIC for confirmation. After the confirmation of the second panel, documentation from both panels will be reviewed by two NPIC designees for:

1. Consistency in identified characteristics of practice within the narratives.
2. Documentation of interview questions and resultant characteristics revealed. A discussion with the two facilitators may be necessary to clarify their respective processes and to enhance growth of facilitation skills. A summary of findings will be forwarded to NPIC.

IX. APPEAL PROCESS

A. The applicant has the option to appeal to a second panel. Application for appeal must be submitted within 30 days of NPIC confirmation. The applicant will submit the same three narratives for the appeal process.
B. The facilitator will know that the panel is an appeal. The members are informed only after they have reached consensus and are strategizing for the interview. No written information from the first panel is shared with the appeal panel in advance.
C. Concerns regarding the CPDM process will be forwarded to the NPIC chairperson or designee immediately.
D. Specialty representation will be present on all appeal panels.
E. Appeals will take priority for scheduling.

X. PANEL NONCONSENSUS

A. If the panel members cannot agree on a recommended stage after the interview, the applicant will be told that the CPDM panel are unable to reach consensus and that a second panel will be scheduled as soon as possible. The second panel will review the same narratives.
B. All efforts will be made to ease this process for the applicant.
C. The NPIC chairperson will be notified immediately.
D. The coach or manager will be notified of the nonconsensus as soon as possible after NPIC notification.

E. Feedback on the characteristics of practice is not to be shared between the first and second panel nor with the coach.

F. Specialty representation is required and present on the second panel.

G. The facilitator of the second panel knows that it is a nonconsensus panel.

H. In the event the second panel is unable to reach consensus re: recommendation of a stage, the facilitator may inform members that this panel is a nonconsensus panel and they too are in nonconsensus. Discuss strategies to inform applicant and NPIC immediately.

XI. FOLLOW-UP AND RECORDS

A. Within one week of NPIC confirmation, the PNA secretary sends congratulatory packet to the manager which includes:
  1. For Applicant
     a. confirmation congratulatory letter
     b. copy of CPDM Panel Staging Summary completed by facilitator
     c. original critique narratives of applicant
     d. CPDM Applicant Feedback form
  2. For Manager (to be placed in unit personnel file)
     a. copy of confirmation congratulatory letter
     b. original CPDM Panel Staging Summary completed by facilitator
  3. For Coach
     a. coach CPDM Feedback Form

B. PNA secretary copies and enters into a computer data base and files any narratives (including panel feedback) which have been identified by facilitators and/or NPIC Chair as potentially useful. The CPDM facilitator recommends narratives that identify new or exemplary characteristics of practice, identify process/systems and /or quality issues and those that would be useful for publication and/or research.

C. NPIC notifies the various PNA Council chairs by sending a form identifying that narratives have been recommended and identified as potentially useful to their council. On a monthly basis copies of narratives would be disseminated to the following councils as appropriate:

NRC/NPC—narratives where characteristics of practice revealed would enhance understanding and/or refinement of the CPDM framework (as identified by facilitator).

NRC—narratives that reveal characteristics of utilizing research in their practice (as identified by facilitator.)

PNRC—narratives approved to be published as identified by (by applicant).

NPIC—narratives that reveal practice or system issues (as identified by facilitator).

XII. Use of Narratives

A. If a PNA Council member or RN (with permission from the Research Council) needs access to narratives, he/she must fill out a PNA narrative agreement form and submit it to the PNA secretary one week before the narratives are needed.

B. In order to maintain anonymity and the confidentiality of narratives the applicant's MRU # will be deleted.

C. The PNA Council member will be notified when the narratives are ready and may come get them after he/she signs them out.

D. Upon completion of the narrative review, the individual must return ALL narratives to the PNA Office so they may be shredded. Narratives should only be signed out for a maximum of one month.

Appendix E

CPDM Applicant Feedback Form

CPDM APPLICANT FEEDBACK FORM

Date:_____
□ SLMC
□ SLSS

You have just completed the CPDM staging/advancement process. The NPIC wants to hear your feedback while the process is fresh in your mind. Please take some time to complete this form now. Seal this form in the enclosed envelope and place it in the NPIC envelope on the interview door. All information is considered confidential.

Thank you,
Nursing Performance Improvement Council

1. Who was your coach?   CNS/NC   Manager   Staff RN
                              □   □   □

2. Did you and your coach have
    one-on-one coaching session(s):   □ yes   □ no
3. To what extent did coaching
    educate and prepare you: Not at all   Greatly
    a) to clarify characteristics of
        practice within the
        CPDM framework   1 2 3 4
    b) to decide for yourself which
        stage to apply   1 2 3 4
    c) for the panel interview process   1 2 3 4
    d) to use strategies for continual growth 1 2 3 4

4. How satisfied were you with the
    following aspects of the coaching
    experience.
                              Not at all satisfied   Greatly satisfied
    a) clarify characteristics of practice
        in relation to the framework   1 2 3 4
    b) help you to decide for which
        stage to apply   1 2 3 4
    c) prepare you for the panel
        interview   1 2 3 4
    d) discuss strategies for your
        continued growth   1 2 3 4

Source: Courtesy of St. Luke's Medical Center, Milwaukee, Wisconsin.

5. Did the interview process give you the
   opportunity to:
   a) talk about your nursing practice   ☐ yes   ☐ no
   b) expand/clarify your narrative   ☐ yes   ☐ no
   c) gain more understanding of the
      CPDM process   ☐ yes   ☐ no
   d) identify areas for continued
      growth in clinical practice   ☐ yes   ☐ no
   e) understand the panel's recom-
      mendation to NPIC for a specific stage   ☐ yes   ☐ no
   f) be treated respectfully by my peers   ☐ yes   ☐ no

6. How satisfied were you with the following
   aspects of the interview experience:

	Not at all satisfied	Greatly satisfied
a) talk about your nursing practice	1 2 3 4	
b) expand/clarify your narrative	1 2 3 4	
c) gain more understanding of the CPDM process	1 2 3 4	
d) understand the panel's recommendation to NPIC for a specific stage	1 2 3 4	
e) be treated respectfully by my peers	1 2 3 4	
f) receive a copy of the CPDM Panel Information form	1 2 3 4	

7. To what extent did the following people support you through your
   CPDM process?

	Not at all	Greatly
Peers	1 2 3 4	
CNS/NC	1 2 3 4	
Manager	1 2 3 4	
Others	1 2 3 4	

8. Do you have any other comments? _____

   _____

   _____

   _____

   _____

Month of Panel Review: Jan. Feb. Mar. April May June July Aug. Sept.
Oct. Nov. Dec.

NAME _____   UNIT: _____   DATE: _____
(Optional)   (Optional)

Thank you for your time. Please seal this form in the enclosed envelope and return to the NPIC envelope on the interview door. All information is considered confidential.

10. Has your nursing practice been affected by the
    CPDM process?   ☐ yes   ☐ no
    a) If yes, please comment _____
       _____
       _____
       _____
       _____
    b) If no, please comment _____
       _____
       _____
       _____
       _____

11. Identify one way in each of the three Domains in which your
    nursing strategies/behaviors have affected patient outcome (re-
    flect on your overall practice, not just the situations in your three
    narratives).

    DOMAINS   PATIENT OUTCOME

    CARING   _____
                                   _____
                                   _____

    CLINICAL KNOWLEDGE/   _____
    DECISION MAKING   _____

    COLLABORATION   _____
                                   _____
                                   _____

Appendix F

CPDM Coach Feedback Form

CPDM COACH FEEDBACK FORM

Date:_____
☐ SLMC
☐ SLSS

Thank you for your participation as coach in the staging/ advancement process of _____, RN. Your feedback is valuable to NPIC in the ongoing monitoring and evaluation of the CPDM process.

1. Did you and the applicant do each of the following:
   a) one-on-one coaching session(s)   ☐ yes ☐ no
   b) discussion of characteristics of practice
      in relation to CPDM framework   ☐ yes ☐ no
   c) discussion about which stage to apply for   ☐ yes ☐ no
   d) preparation for interview   ☐ yes ☐ no
   e) discussion of strategies for continued
      growth   ☐ yes ☐ no

2. To what degree were you and the applicant in agreement regarding stage and characteristics of practice by the end of the coaching session(s)?
   Very Little   1   2   3   4   Very Much
   Comments:

3. How much consistency was there between your identification of characteristics of practice and those identified by the panel? (Written feedback on narratives or as reported by applicant.)
   Very Little   1   2   3   4   Very Much
   Comments:

4. What was the recognition/celebration with this applicant after completion of the staging/advancement process?

5. Do you have any comments or concerns regarding the process with this applicant?

Name: _____ Unit: _____ Date: _____
Thank you for your time. Please send to: **NPIC Chairperson**
                                            PNA Office
                                            SLMC

Source: Courtesy of St. Luke's Medical Center, Milwaukee, Wisconsin.

Index

Collaborative governance structure, Massachusetts General Hospital, 199–202
Compensation, issues related to, 153–154
Competent nurse
  characteristics of, 54, 56–57, 60
  job description, 154–155
Coordination of care
  nurse as coordinator, 161–162
  Outcome Facilitation Teams, 162–163
Culture, effects on patient care, 9

D

Debriefing, research bias protection, 219–220
Decision making, and clinical knowledge, 51, 56–57
Dependability, research, 221, 225
Developmental model, versus career ladder, 44
Diversity Steering Committee, role of, 201
Domains, 49, 50–52
Dreyfus Model of Skill Acquisition, 53, 54–55

E

Educational activities
  expert nurses, 191
  narratives, 77–78
  post–implementation, 77
  See also Coaching
Ethics in Clinical Practice Committee, role of, 201

Experiential learning, and clinical knowledge, 26, 37–39
Expert nurses
  characteristics of, 49–52, 56–57, 60
  and coordination of care, 161–162
  education activities, 191
  narrative of, 58–59, 62–63
  research activities, 191
External validity, research, 220–221

F

Facilitators
  qualifications of, 106
  role expectations, 106–107
  role of, 102, 104–107, 113–114
Family Practice Center, 157
  resident teaching program, 157
Feedback forms, 169, 276–280
Fittingness, research, 220–221
Functional councils, Professional Nursing Assembly, 247

G

Governance. *See* Shared governance
Governing councils, Professional Nursing Assembly, 247

H

Hiring process, 156–157
Holistic approach, meaning of, 14
House–wide panels, 102–104

About the Contributors

Barbara Haag-Heitman, RN, MSN, CS was a Clinical Nurse Specialist at St. Luke's Medical Center at the time of the development of the Clinical Practice Development Model. She is currently working in the Women's Health Product Line in the Milwaukee area for parent company Aurora Healthcare.

Patricia Benner, RN, PhD, FAAN is Professor of Nursing in the Department of Physiological Nursing at the University of California, San Francisco, School of Nursing. Dr. Benner is the author of *From Novice to Expert: Excellence and Power in Clinical Nursing Practice* Published by Addision-Wesley, which has won the AJN Book of the Year Award and has been translated into eight languages. Most recently she co-authored *Expertise in Nursing Practice, Caring, Clinical Judgement and Ethics* with Christine Tanner and Catherine Chesla (Springer Publishers), and *Clinical Wisdom in Critical Care: A Thinking-in-Action Approach* with Patricia Hooper-Kyriakidis and Daphne Stannard. She served as a consultant on the Clinical Practice Development Model.

Richard V. Benner, PhD is president of Benner Associates, an organizational development consulting firm, and has been a lecturer in organizational behavior at the Haas School of Business at the University of California, where he was Assistant Dean for ten years. He has degrees in philosophy, counseling psychology, and received his doctorate from Stanford University in organizational studies where his dissertation on decision making in complex organizations received a national award. He was lead consultant for the Clinical Practice Development Model at St. Luke's Medical Center and a regional model.

Laura J. Burke, PhD, RN, FAAN was a Special Research Projects Coordinator at the time of the model development. She facilitated the research related to staff nurse attitudes toward transition. She is now the Director of Nursing Research for the Metro Region of Aurora Health Care and consulted on the validity and reliability of the metro model.

Carol Camooso, RN, MS is a Professional Development Coordinator in the Center for Clinical and Professional Development at Massachusetts General Hospital. As coach of the Professional Development Committee, she is supporting the work of the disciplines within Patient Care Services as they design an advancement program for clinicians. Carol is also working with clinicians and leadership in their utilization of clinical narratives as tools to enhance professional development.

Theresa Dirienzo, RN, BSN was a member of the Quality Council at the time of development and implementation of the Clinical Practice Development Model. She became the chairperson of that council shortly after the transition. She is a staff nurse in the Preadmissions Test Center and a facilitator and panel member for the peer review process.

Jeanne Smrz DuPont, RN, BSN is a staff nurse in the Emergency Department at St. Luke's Medical Center. She participated in the development of Clinical Practice Development Model and is a facilitator/panel member for the peer review process. She is also responsible for training new panel members and facilitators.

Marie P. Farrell, EdD, RN, MPH holds the Walter Schroeder Chair and is a Professor of Nursing Research, jointly appointed between the University of Wisconsin-School of Nursing and Aurora HealthCare-Metro Region. She is a nurse researcher for Aurora HealthCare.

Vicki George, RN, MSN, PhD was the Chief Nurse Executive and Vice President for Nursing at St. Luke's at the time of the model development and implementation. She is currently the Chief Nurse Executive for the Metro Region of Aurora Healthcare.

Sharon Gray, RN, BSN is a Nurse Clinician on an orthopedic/surgical unit at Sinai Samaritan Medical Center in Milwaukee. She participated in the design and implementation of the Metro Clinical Practice Development Model, a regional developmental model.

Alice Kramer, RN, MS is a Clinical Nurse Specialist in Emergency Services at St. Luke's Medical Center. She was involved in the development and implementation of both St. Luke's Clinical Practice Development Model and a Regional Model. She also mentors others in the coaching role.

Nora Ladewig, RN, MSN was the President of the Professional Nursing Assembly and staff nurse in the Surgical/Neuro Intensive Care Unit at the time of development and implementation of the Clinical Practice Development Model. In this role, she served as the Chairperson of the Steering Committee that guided the implementation process and at the completion of her term of office, served as a peer review panel member for five years. She is currently a Clinical Nurse Specialist working at St. Luke's Medical Center.

Sue Luedtke, RN, MSN is the Patient Care Manager on a Surgical Cardiac Unit at St. Luke's Medical Center. She was a member of the Narrative Workgroup that developed the Clinical Practice Development Model and a member of the Management Council at the time of the implementation.

Susan A. Nuccio, RN, MSN was the chairperson of the Research Council Workgroup responsible for evaluating the transition process of the CPDM Model. Presently she is a clinical nurse specialist at St. Luke's Medical Center.

Julie Raaum, RN, MS was a staff nurse working in the Surgical/Neuro Intensive Care Unit at the time of development and implementation of the Clinical Practice Development Model. She was chairperson for the Quality Council during the transition and participated on the peer review panels. She is currently a Family Nurse Practitioner and working in Milwaukee.